Back to Life, Back to Normality

Cognitive Therapy, Recovery and Psychosis

Douglas Turkington, David Kingdon,
Shanaya Rathod, Sarah K. J. Wilcock,
Alison Brabban, Paul Cromarty,
Robert Dudley, Richard Gray, Jeremy Pelton,
Ron Siddle, Peter Weiden

Foreword by

Aaron T. Beck

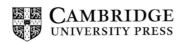
UNIVERSITY PRESS

CAMBRIDGE UNIVERSITY PRESS
Cambridge, New York, Melbourne, Madrid, Cape Town, Singapore, São Paulo, Delhi

Cambridge University Press
The Edinburgh Building, Cambridge CB2 8RU, UK

Published in the United States of America by Cambridge University Press, New York

www.cambridge.org
Information on this title: www.cambridge.org/9780521699563

First published 2009

Printed in the United Kingdom at the University Press, Cambridge

A catalogue record for this publication is available from the British Library

ISBN 978-0-521-69956-3 paperback

Back to Life, Back to Normality

Cognitive Therapy, R

Contents

Foreword

Cognitive therapy (CT) of psychotic disorders such as schizophrenia has grown and developed dramatically over the last ten years. In the UK, the National Institute for Health and Clinical Excellence (NICE, 2002) recommends that CT should be made available for all people suffering with schizophrenia, particularly those with persistent hallucinations and delusions, lack of insight, and poor concordance with antipsychotic medication. However, the interest in cognitive therapy for psychosis goes beyond the UK. The USA, Canada, the Netherlands, and Australia have well-developed research programs in this area and Brazil, China, Germany, Japan, Scandinavia, and Spain are all showing an increasing interest in this approach.

Unfortunately, despite growing interest, access to CT by people suffering from psychosis is limited largely due to a shortage of suitably trained therapists. Now, this current volume by Turkington and colleagues attempts to bridge this gap by providing guidance on self-management of psychosis. Written specifically with psychosis sufferers and carers in mind, the book allows those experiencing psychosis and their carers to understand and apply the basic concepts of CT for psychosis.

The book contains many nuggets of commonsense wisdom, which, when applied, will begin to help. Until now carers, friends, colleagues, and those suffering with psychotic symptoms have only really had the option of referring to psychiatric textbooks to try to find out how to help themselves or their loved ones with psychosis. This book provides a straightforward and practical guide for carers, helping them know what to say and what to do. The book aims to increase their understanding of how the psychosis started and also which factors worsen symptoms or increase the likelihood of relapse. They will also learn how to help symptoms settle and delay or prevent relapse. This text illustrates how common psychosis is and how people's lives can be restored using CT.

In addition, this book provides an excellent resource for mental health professionals working with patients with schizophrenia. Not only can this book be used to support ongoing cognitive therapy of psychosis, but it can also be used by clinicians working in a variety of settings who wish to introduce patients to this approach prior to a trained cognitive therapist being allocated. This book can be used by mental health professionals as needed, even in briefer appointment settings. Single chapters can be given to individuals experiencing psychosis and can be worked through systematically. There is space for self-reflection and comment, with exercises to help sufferers understand their symptoms, explore their own beliefs and feelings, and reflect on the way they cope.

I am proud to give this book my personal endorsement. The authors have long experience of CT for psychosis and have now written a text to make that experience available to all.

Aaron T. Beck, M.D.
University Professor of Psychiatry
University of Pennsylvania
Department of Psychiatry
Philadelphia, PA, USA

REFERENCES

National Institute for Health and Clinical Excellence (2002). Clinical Guideline 1. Schizophrenia: core interventions in the treatment and management of schizophrenia in primary and secondary care. London: NICE.

Acknowledgments

We would like primarily to acknowledge all those currently experiencing psychosis for all they have taught us. We acknowledge those carers and friends who have for so long shown such patience and dignity with mental health services that have not always recognized their potential role as co-workers on the road to recovery from psychosis. We acknowledge the work of Marius Romme and Sandra Escher who started the move towards the destigmatizing of psychosis through the establishment of the Hearing Voices Network.

Beck's breakthrough in cognitive therapy (CT) was elaborated and more fully applied to patients with psychotic symptoms by the British School. Simultaneously, in the early 1990s several British investigators developed viable cognitive models and effective interventions based on the principles of CT. Acknowledgments need to go to the following: Birmingham (including Max Brichwood, Val Drury, and Peter Trower), East Anglia (David Fowler), Glasgow (Andrew Gumley), Liverpool (Richard Bentall, Peter Kinderman), London (Daniel Freeman, Phillipa Garety, Elizabeth Kuipers, Craig Steel, Emmanuel Peters), Manchester (Christine Barrowclough, Paul French, Gillian Haddock, Tony Morrison, Nick Tarrier), Newcastle (Pauline Calcott, Steve Moorhead, Jan Scott), Southampton (Paul Chadwick).

On the international stage the following cognitive therapists have established CT for psychosis services and research programs within their own domains. We acknowledge their vision and energy. In Australia, Pat McGorry, Alison Jung, and Paddy Power integrated CT in their early intervention programs. In Brazil, Anna Maria Serra has set up CT of psychosis training workshops. In Canada, Jean Addington in Toronto has manualized CT for Early Intervention services, Neil Rector has worked on the CT of negative symptoms, and Tania Lecompte has developed and researched a manualized group program. In China, Dr. Li of Capitol University is running a randomized controlled trial of psychiatrists using CT with patients with schizophrenia. In Germany, Tania Lincoln is researching CT for psychosis. In Italy, Antonio Pinto described the benefits of CT when combined with clozapine. In the Netherlands, Mark Van Der Gaag has designed and researched CT interventions for psychosis. In the USA, Neil

Stollar is working to integrate biological and cognitive models. Corinne Cather, David Penn, Eric Granholm, Yulia Landa, Paul Grant, Page Burkholder, and Mike Garrett are progressing the understanding and practice of CT for psychosis in their own centers.

We acknowledge the work of all those mental health professionals who have for so long, and often in isolation, struggled to improve the lot of their psychotic patients. Hopefully this text will help to support their work.

Finally, we must acknowledge the father of CT, who has been an inspiration to us all: Aaron T. Beck, who in 1952 wrote the original paper describing the successful treatment of a patient with paranoia using CT. Dr. Beck continues to take a leading role in progressing the practice of CT for psychosis, integrating these strands of research in his annual CT of psychosis conference.

REFERENCES

Beck, A.T. (1952). Successful outpatient psychotherapy of a chronic schizophrenic patient with a delusion based on borrowed guilt. *Psychiatry*, **15**, 305–12.

About the authors

Douglas Turkington is a psychiatrist working in Newcastle, UK. He works with the Liaison Psychiatry Service at the Royal Victoria Infirmary for Northumberland, Tyne and Wear NHS Trust. He is also Professor of Psychosocial Psychiatry at Newcastle University.

David Kingdon is a community psychiatrist working in Southampton, UK. He holds the chair of Mental Health Care Delivery at the University of Southampton.

Shanaya Rathod is a consultant psychiatrist in general adult psychiatry and is also Associate Medical Director of the Mid Hants and Eastleigh Locality of the Hampshire Partnership NHS Trust, UK.

Sarah K. J. Wilcock is a senior practitioner with the Assertive Outreach Team of Tees, Esk and Wear Valleys NHS Trust based in Redcar, Cleveland, UK. She works with people suffering severe and enduring mental illnesses, their relatives, and carers.

Alison Brabban is a clinical psychologist with the Early Intervention in Psychosis Team within Tees, Esk and Wear Valleys NHS Trust in the North East of England, UK.

Paul Cromarty is Course Director of the CBT course at the University of Cumbria, UK and Honorary Clinical Specialist at Newcastle Cognitive and Behavioural Therapies Centre.

Robert Dudley is a psychologist and team leader with the South of Tyne Early Intervention in Psychosis Team based in Sunderland, UK.

Richard Gray is a mental health nurse working in Norwich, UK. He is Professor of Nursing Related to Research at the University of East Anglia.

Jeremy Pelton is a nurse manager at Innovex Health Management Services, UK.

Ron Siddle is a psychologist and clinical lead of the Early Interventions Service at Cumbria Partnership NHS Foundation Trust.

Peter Weiden is head of schizophrenia research at the University of Chicago, IL, USA.

Introduction

Douglas Turkington and Peter Weiden

"I actually looked forward to the CBT sessions and talking about my symptoms."
(A service user with severe paranoia)

What is psychosis?

Psychosis, neurosis, and normality all lie on a spectrum. In psychotic disorders, patients experience symptoms such as hearing voices that no one else can hear or believing things that others believe to be false. In psychosis there is difficulty in thinking and concentrating, and often problems with motivation. Social functioning such as self-care, friendships, and work often deteriorate without treatment.

What is recovery?

Over the medium term the outcome for psychosis is reasonably good. Recovery involves learning to overcome symptoms, to reach the very best level of social performance that can be achieved for any individual.

Why have we written this book?

In the year 2000, six mental health nurses were trained to use cognitive behavioral therapy techniques (CBT) for patients with severe nervous breakdowns (schizophrenia). The nurses went out into community mental health teams and used CBT for 257 patients with psychotic symptoms. Carers were also trained how to use CBT at home. The main finding from this study was that this new way of working was very much appreciated by patients and carers alike. The general feedback was that people with psychosis often felt very isolated, and often they had only medication and occasional supportive visits before the CBT sessions started. Users and carers had so many questions that they wanted to ask, but there had simply never been the time before. The CBT nurse initially spent time listening to the patient's and carer's points of view and beliefs about what was going on in their lives, and often new and sometimes useful insights were arrived at. Thereafter the CBT nurse used normalizing to explain that anyone can have these frightening experiences, e.g., in some surveys one person in five had experienced recent paranoid thoughts. It was also explained that severe symptoms can improve, and that we can often work out what is keeping them going and then do something about it. The nurses tried to help patients engage and test out frightening symptoms, such as voices and beliefs of persecution. They then tried to make sense of the medication situation, improve self-esteem, and work out a relapse prevention plan. All the sessions were based on a "working together" approach, with both nurse and user doing some homework to try and investigate things further. Many patients felt that this way of investigating things together was the best form of help they had ever received. Many described success in fighting off unpleasant experiences and feelings, leading to a more active and fulfilling life.

"It was the first time someone had sat down with me and focused on my problems." (Service user)

Carers were equally enthusiastic as they felt that they understood the psychotic symptoms better and knew how to say and do helpful things. It must be said that carers were often initially angry at what they perceived as a lack of instruction as to how to help their relative who was suffering so desperately with these frightening symptoms.

"How come this service has never been available before?" (Irate carer)

The CBT nurse could only agree about the lack of psychoeducation and family therapy in many areas and use CBT to reduce carer stress, and then start to develop a CBT strategy to help their relative. Carers often had automatic thoughts in the back of their minds as follows.[1]

Common carer automatic thoughts

"This is my fault."
"I did something wrong in childhood."
"I am a bad mother/father."

---

[1] The term automatic thought refers to the first thought that comes into your mind when presented with a piece of information. This thought can often be of a negative nature.

Or

"I'm going to make them see sense and pull themselves out of this."
"They just need to find a good job."
"How dare they not take the medicine . . . it obviously helps."

If you are a carer then enter your automatic thoughts about your situation here:

1.

2.

3.

Both sets of thoughts lead to carers experiencing stress and exhaustion. The first set of thoughts cause sadness and anxiety in a carer, and often they end up doing too much for their relative. The second set of thoughts cause frustration and anger, and lead to a carer "overdoing it" in trying to force their relative back to health. Carers often have both sets of thoughts. Both sets of thoughts are distorted and can be corrected. The first set is too self-blaming and a good rational response (corrected thinking style) is "no one knows the cause of this illness, but it happens in every country in the world"; "any human person can have a breakdown . . . it's usually caused by a combination of genetics, personality, and stress"; "I'm still an OK parent." Similarly, for the angry thoughts the antidote for the thinking would be "too much pressure obviously doesn't help"; "we need to go slowly but steadily"; "I can back off a bit and try a different approach." Reducing carer stress in this way really helps to improve the atmosphere at home and can pave the way for further progress. Psychiatrists also suffer from these stressful thoughts. I have just had the thought pop into my mind that if I stayed up very late I could finish this chapter tonight. I felt a bit tense and a bit down because it is a big job. I used CBT to tell myself "you are having those workaholic thoughts again. Three pages a day will finish it in two weeks, and it will be better in quality" – I immediately felt less stressed as I knew I was right . . . a rushed chapter would be a less good chapter. In this way we can get to know our minds and the way they cause and handle stress. All users should also have a think about whether they feel stressed, and if so try to write the thoughts down in the space below.

1.

2.

3.

User example: *"I'm scared to stay in and scared to go out."*
Carer example: *"She's bone idle."*

Automatic thoughts are usually distorted ... are the thoughts on page 3 correct or can we correct them?

Magnification (making things seem worse than they really are).

Labeling (putting a global label on a person).

Examples of corrected thoughts:

User: *"Well I suppose I have not been attacked in the last number of months. Maybe at least I am safe in the house."*

Carer: *"My daughter is still recovering from a severe breakdown and has some medication side effects. She used to be a good worker–perhaps we can slowly get there again."*

The effect of this more rational thinking in the home is of improved optimism and reduced argument. From this point on, plans for future progress need to be jointly agreed and worked on together.

Try to write corrected thoughts below and then keep bringing these thoughts back to mind from time to time. Do you feel a bit easier?

1.

2.

Psychiatrists are not hostile to the idea of patients and carers being guided through CBT. Cognitive behavioral therapy is a therapy supportive of using antipsychotic medication, in a dose that is jointly agreed between user and psychiatrist. Although there can be side effects with antipsychotic medication, there is definite protection against relapse as well as real benefits for many patients in relation to distressing hallucinations, delusions, and thinking difficulties. Cognitive behavioral therapy also endorses the use of clozapine,[2] which can at times be very effective when other drugs have failed. Cognitive behavioral therapy can also be combined with group therapy and family therapy. It is, however, different from psychoeducation and psychoanalysis, and these should not be done at the same time as CBT or there might be a risk of some confusion. Please tell your psychiatrist or case manager that you wish to work with this book before you proceed, so that they can advise you how to use the book. The following are statements made by consultant psychiatrists who have had experience of CBT being delivered to patients with schizophrenia in their area of the UK.

"The CBT nurse has highlighted the need for making use of CBT skills ... we would like to have someone as an integral part of the team. CBT has helped keep people out of hospital." (Croydon)

---

[2] Clozapine is an antipsychotic medication.

"It has been very beneficial to staff and patients working with the CBT nurse. Our team has learned a lot and patients have clearly enjoyed and moved on following the programme." (Edinburgh)

"CBT is delivered in a professional, dynamic, and realistic fashion." (Liverpool)

"Most patients are much improved by CBT, and a demand from patients and carers has been created. Very positive for the Trust." (Leicester)

So, if patients and carers do invest time and energy in following the exercises in this book what can they expect? The vast majority of people derive some benefit and many derive a lot of benefit. The first thing is that by practicing these techniques they become less stressed and more optimistic. Nerves and sadness, which are almost always present in a severe nervous breakdown, can improve. Other symptoms, such as voices and paranoia, can often become more manageable as patients and carers understand them better and find new ways of dealing with them. As such there can be an improvement in insight leading to better coping, improved activity levels and relationships, and an improved overall quality of life. These effects, however, do not occur overnight; they usually develop slowly following a period of joint work. One of the most important effects of CBT is to prevent or delay relapse. In those who do relapse following CBT it tends to take longer, i.e., patients stay well longer. Also, in those who do relapse, having learned the new understandings and techniques of CBT they can tend to work their way out of hospital more quickly, i.e., they spend less time hospitalized. The effects on relapse and hospitalization on their own would be very well worth having, but CBT offers much more than this. On the down side one person in ten doesn't really like CBT, but it is a safe treatment, which doesn't lead to suicide or any dangerous side effects. As with any such treatment it is important not to rush at it like a bull in a china shop, but to do the exercises properly one at a time with the help of others and in particular your mental health worker and/or carer.

Why write this book now?

This is the ideal time to publish a book about CBT for severe mental health problems. An important government body (the National Institute for Health and Clinical Excellence, NICE) has examined all the evidence for different forms of treatment for schizophrenia. It has decided that atypical anti-psychotics are to be made available,[3] as well as rapid access to clozapine if

---

[3] "Atypical" is a term used that refers to a newer form of antipsychotic that has fewer side effects than older drugs known as "typical" antipsychotics.

needed. It has also stressed the importance of psychoeducation, family therapy, work opportunities, and the need for a more optimistic "recovery" perspective. It made a strong statement about CBT. Cognitive behavioral therapy is to be made available for every patient in the UK with schizophrenia, but in particular for those with persistent symptoms, poor compliance with medication, and lack of insight. By persistent symptoms, NICE meant all symptoms such as hallucinations, delusions, thinking problems, anxiety, sadness, etc., which don't clear up with medication treatment. The National Institute for Health and Clinical Excellence has published its findings in a clinical guideline, which has been sent to the chief executive of every Mental Health Trust and Primary Care Trust in the UK. Chief executives have been given the role of implementing the guideline in their trusts and this will be audited. Because of this, many mental health workers are learning the CBT techniques outlined in this book. Cognitive behavioral therapy is often taught in psychosocial interventions schemes (PSI) or in specific brief courses on CBT for hallucinations, delusions, and negative symptoms. There should be, within the not-too-distant future, a local worker who can help you to work your way through this book. The book will be useful as a means of structuring the CBT sessions, so please tell your key worker about the book and ask for guidance and support. Finding practical, simple solutions to help with troublesome symptoms may only be a few pages away.

Family therapy has been recommended for situations where there is a lot of distress in the family and the patient is relapsing regularly. However, the majority of carers do not require a full intensive family therapy approach. Most carers want to understand more about the roots of the psychosis, about the factors that prevent it from settling down, and about the things that they can say and do that will be most helpful. This book is for them.

One caveat: if a user wishes to read this book without guidance that is OK, but the book is best used with help from a mental health professional. Some of the techniques do need explaining, and sometimes things can get slightly worse before they get better so do find someone to share with.

Who else is this book written for?

- Patients, carers, and friends who want to know some simple things that they can do to help.
- Mental health professionals in training (psychiatrists, psychologists, mental health nurses, social workers, and occupational therapists) as a primer and as a homework book.
- For use in groups, e.g., day hospital, rehabilitation, Hearing Voices, Rethink, MIND, when there is a group leader with knowledge of CBT for psychosis.

Why CBT for severe mental disorders?

- Cognitive behavioral therapy is the best researched therapy for patients with schizophrenia and other linked psychoses. This is not to say that other forms of individual therapy (e.g., supportive therapy, counselling, personal therapy, or interpersonal therapy) do not work. It's just that we know that we are on safe ground with CBT as it has been so widely researched.
- It is easy to learn, flexible, and safe.
- In 1952, using this method, Dr. Aaron T. Beck helped a man with severe paranoia (105 suspected persecutors) to become much less frightened and to lead a much improved life.
- Since then, 22 proper scientific studies have confirmed that CBT really helps in persistent symptoms, particularly hallucinations and delusions.

What do the CBT therapists really think of CBT?

- Cognitive behavioral therapy is used by all those who have learned it, to help themselves and their friends if troubled.
- I used to be very frightened about speaking in public, now I give lectures all the time. I discovered thoughts in my mind that the audience were thinking: "what a bore ... this talk stinks ... he looks bad ... he should shut up and get off."
- My anxiety only reduced when I asked people directly what they thought of my lecture. To my surprise they were quite positive. I had to keep telling myself that I was OK and to keep going.
- With practice my confidence improved, and I started to enjoy the lectures and make them humorous and creative. My anxiety reduced. Anxiety is very often an important part of keeping paranoia and voices at a distressingly high level.
- Road rage is another good example. A man driving a car sees another man pull out directly in front of him almost causing an accident. The first driver gets very angry and rushes out of the car to attack the other driver only to notice that the driver's wife is giving birth in the back seat. There was no insult intended. The first driver got it wrong. Anger is often like that – it can worsen voices and paranoia; however, it can be reduced by checking things out as in this example. So we want to use CBT to reduce the unpleasant and unhelpful emotions of anxiety and anger.

The simple cognitive model is that we all think about the things happening in our life, and these thoughts are sometimes too extreme or not based on fact. If we change the thoughts we can feel better and do things differently. The more we do this, the better we feel.

So how can CBT help severe problems?

In much the same way, by improving understanding and using CBT to reduce distress and then by finding strategies that work to improve things.

These are some signals that indicate that you could be helped by CBT:

- voices and delusions
- strong emotions (anger, anxiety, shame, sadness)
- hiding away from the world
- getting into lots of arguments with others
- not thinking clearly
- not looking after yourself well, or not having any drive to do things.

If any of the above apply to you then working through the relevant sections of this book could be useful. Remember to read through the book slowly a page at a time and do the exercises suggested. They are not usually difficult or challenging and are best done when you can check the findings out with another person. You can jump straight to the most relevant chapter if you are very keen to get started and make some progress, but we would recommend reading through the explanations chapter, at least, before moving on to other sections. With all CBT, practice is the key ... the benefits build up gradually.

So why haven't people been using CBT for ages? It seems so obvious!

People who are suffering with a severe nervous breakdown with the above symptoms tend not to investigate things, or try enough things to fight back. Often they believe there is an incurable madness there, but the studies show that people can improve a lot. Much of this is down to society's attitudes to mental illness. People often just don't want to know if you're a voice hearer, or a bit paranoid, or have lost your drive. Then there is the label of schizophrenia, which has all kinds of negative connotations. People still think of schizophrenia as "multiple personality" (i.e., Jekyll and Hyde), which is a frightening idea. People also still have the old biblical idea of demon possession. Both of these common stereotypes are complete myths! Then there are the common stories in the newspapers about people with schizophrenia or paranoia being violent. This is actually extremely rare, but the media and news broadcast seems to always make a point of reporting it in a very sensational way.

What are your own automatic thoughts about your breakdown?

Perhaps you have thoughts like the ones above, which are making you feel stigmatized or ashamed?

User thoughts about schizophrenia/paranoia and psychiatry

Example: *"People with schizophrenia have nothing to offer and might as well give up."* (Emotion: sadness and despair)

Response: *"Johnny Nash fully recovered and is a university professor!"* (Emotion: some optimism and a bit of determination!)

Put your own and your carer's automatic thoughts about mental illness below:
1.

2.

3.

Now the rational responses:
1.

2.

3.

Discuss these new ideas with friends, other users, etc. Consider writing a short letter about the subject, and send it to a local magazine or newspaper.

Cultural and religious aspects

It is common to think that a therapy like CBT "does not apply to me if I am from a particular cultural or religious background" or "what do they understand about my culture/religion?" Sometimes this assumption may be true, as every therapist does not understand every culture or religion. But CBT is not about challenging cultural or religious beliefs in a way that seems disrespectful. It is about understanding perspectives in order to ease the distress associated with symptoms such as voices or paranoid thoughts. The same assumptions apply to carers who may feel that "if I ask for support, it may sound like I am complaining – culturally, it is my duty to care." It is not the intention of the therapist to judge carers about their role and culture. The aim is to improve understanding and support the carers.

Every chapter in this book has a section on cultural and religious aspects, which shows how the process can be modified and applied to everyone. Do you have any worries that professionals may misunderstand you due to their lack of understanding of your culture or religion? Please list them:

1.

2.

3.

Discuss these with a therapist or a senior figure from your faith.

Who is this book for exactly?

- If you have been told that you have a severe nervous breakdown such as psychosis, schizophrenia, schizoaffective disorder, delusional disorder, or even psychotic depression this book may really help.
- It is important to realize that anyone can suffer in the way that you are suffering, and that you are not alone ... paranoid ideas are found in some 20% of the population and 15% of people hear voices at some point in their life. It may be helpful to join a support group – ask your therapist or local mental health voluntary group for details.
- The key message here is that something can be done and the more that you engage with your symptoms, your situation, and your life the more you can move toward better control and more satisfaction in relation to your life goals.

This book complements:

- taking good quality medication at the right dose
- family therapy
- community psychiatry
- rehabilitation
- employment placements
- always check with your consultant/key worker or primary care physician that it is a good idea in your present circumstances.

Summary

To get the most from this book, it would be best to complete the questions in this introduction before you move on to Chapter 1. Remember, Rome wasn't built in a day! Take your time, think things over, and keep trying these ideas out ... you will begin to change for the better!

Where do I begin? (...or so many problems, so little time!)

Jeremy Pelton

Overview

This chapter aims to offer the reader guidance in how to begin the process of understanding what is wrong with them. It suggests how the road to recovery might be found and how to begin to walk along that path. Simple CBT techniques are described to help you start to take control of your life again.

Chapter contents

- Personal example
- Diaries
- Stress
- Functioning
- Symptoms
- Timelines
- Case studies
- Cultural and religious aspects
- Summary

"It's not what happens to you, but how you react to it that matters." (Epictetus (AD 55–AD 135) Stoic philosopher)

Where do I begin? This is often the 64 million dollar question! By the time you are asking the question there can be so much going on that it's very hard to put things into perspective and make sense of what is happening. Psychosis is a complex condition and trying to put a finger on when the first episode began, or even when the latest episode started, can be extremely difficult. It is often insidious: an experience that creeps up on you unexpectedly. The earlier you or a relative/friend notices the signs, the easier it is to do something about it.

Personal example

There are times at work when I feel that everything is starting to get on top of me, because there is so much happening and deadlines appear from nowhere. This is often an experience that builds up over a number of days or weeks, and it sometimes takes a while for either myself, my manager, or my family to notice. However, if it is noticed earlier on, I find it so much easier to nip it in the bud and can use a number of techniques such as diary planning, prioritizing events, and time management to alleviate my problems.

This chapter will look at explanations and exercises that will help you identify what you are experiencing and to understand what the experiences may be and why they are happening. There will then be further chapters throughout this book that will help you deal with these experiences. Every one of us has different experiences that are personal to us, and we all respond to these experiences in a way that is individual to us.

This is a normal process that takes into account: firstly, how we have developed as an individual; and secondly, what environmental factors we have around us at any given time. We can take these one at a time and explore them further.

- Organic factors. If there is a strong family history of mental illness there may be genes that make you more vulnerable to psychosis at times of stress. These are inherited factors. Similarly, if the brain has been exposed to hypoxia at the time of birth this can affect the areas of the brain involved with speech and belief formation.
- Development factors. These can be any experiences from a person's childhood and adolescence (formative years) that affect how we develop and mature. They include, among others, relationships (both family and friends) and childhood experiences.
- Environmental factors. These are the everyday occurrences/stresses that are going on in your life in the here and now. They include, among others: relationships (both family and friends), finances, accommodation, vocational and social activities.

The organic and development factors are less easy to alter or modify compared to the environmental ones, and with this in mind, and for the purpose of the chapter, we will be concentrating on the latter.

Diaries

A good starting point of "where do I begin?" is to keep a diary, as writing things down in an organized, structured way can be a useful step in making sense of our experiences. Seeing a diary page in black and white in front of you is a lot easier to understand than having everything racing around in your head. There are a number of diary templates available through mental health professionals and the internet. One format that has proven useful with many of the people I have worked with is to fill in the template below (see Template A).

Template A

Date: **Time:**

Event (What was happening?)

Thought (What was I thinking?)

Emotion (How was I feeling?)

Behavior (What did I do?)

At the end of each day put aside half an hour, either by yourself or with a relative or friend, and list two or three significant events from that day.

This is a good opportunity to involve someone else in this process. The mere fact that you are discussing your experiences with another person will help you. It will also help that person come to an understanding of what you are experiencing. This will be a little strange at first, but start to plan this time into your day and allow it to become a routine.

It may help to keep a pencil and paper with you during the day so that you can make notes as and when the event occurs – it is amazing how quickly we can forget details around an event.

Enter each event into its own template and think about or discuss your thoughts, feelings, and actions. Have a look at the example below to guide you (see Example 1).

Example 1

> **Date:** November 11, 2007 **Time:** 10 am
>
> **Event** (What was happening?)
> *I was walking through the local shopping mall when I noticed a man in a black jacket looking at me.*
> **Thought** (What was I thinking?)
> *He knows me and is going to attack me.*
> **Affect** (How was I feeling?)
> *Anxious/worried/afraid.*
> **Behavior** (What did I do?)
> *I put my head down and walked home as fast as I could.*

By filling in the template you are starting to formulate your experience and begin the process of making sense of it. In the example given the event has been recorded and the person has had a chance to think about it and record their thoughts, feelings, and behavior. Also the thought might occur "Could I have been jumping to conclusions about the man? Maybe he was just looking at my new baseball cap."

Stress

As I mentioned at the beginning of the chapter "Every one of us has different experiences that are personal to us, and we all respond to these experiences in a way that is individual to each of us." So you could ask six people who have experienced the same event as described above and they could all record different responses as to their thoughts, feelings, and behaviors. **This is normal**.

What we also know from working with people with similar experiences, is that when we take into account that person's environmental factors it is possible that they could experience the same event three or four times in a month and record different responses to their thoughts, feelings, and behaviors each time.

If a person has a number of environmental factors not going their way at any point in time, this can cause them to react to an event in a different way. **Again, this is normal.**

For example, look at the two scenarios below and the factors associated with each; assuming that they are the same person, but on a different day, how are they going to react to a similar event? Can you think of similar examples yourself?

Scenario A: Pear shaped	Scenario B: Hunky dory
• Big argument with wife • Bad night's sleep • Big bill arrived that morning • Forgot to pick up prescription and had missed last two days of medication	• Good relationship with wife • Good night's sleep • Small lottery win • Medication taken as prescribed
Worried/anxious/concerned	*Feeling good about themselves*

Most people who are faced with Scenario A compared to Scenario B are going to be more vulnerable to events, as they have a number of environmental factors not going their way, and these factors are going to lead to a certain amount of stress.

Using the blank template below, think about the factors that affect you and list what is going on in your life on a typical good day, compared to what may change on what you would define as a typical bad day. (See Template B below.)

Template B

Scenario A: Bad day	Scenario B: Good day

This is something else you can record when completing your diary. Firstly, list your two or three events and the associated thoughts, feelings, and behavior, and then for that day give your level of stress a percentage rating. Think of your personal environmental factors: 0% is no stress at all and 100% is the worst stress you have experienced (see Example 2, self-disclosure).

Example 2

Date: November 12, 2007 **Time:** 10 pm **Stress:** 75%
Event (What was happening?)
I was lying in bed when I started to see faces coming out of the wall.
Thought (What was I thinking?)
What is happening, am I going mad?
Affect (How was I feeling?)
Scared.
Behavior (What did I do?)
I got out of bed and went downstairs.

You will now have begun a diary where you are not only recording the events and your thoughts, feelings, and behaviors for that day, but also your level of stress at that point in time. As the diary builds and you have a number of records in front of you, there will be a chance to analyze and look for patterns linked to your levels of stress but also to your thoughts, feelings, and behaviors.

Functioning

The next step can be to look at the *consequence* of your thoughts, feelings, and behaviors. In Example 1, the person may repeatedly have this experience of feeling that someone is watching him in the local shopping mall – this may get to a point where the person only goes to the shopping mall when it is very quiet and therefore he is less likely to see people watching him. Or, worse still, he avoids the shopping mall completely.

Example 1

Date: November 11, 2007 **Time:** 10 am
Event (What was happening?)
I was walking through the local shopping mall when I noticed a man in a black jacket looking at me.
Thought (What was I thinking?)
He knows me and is going to attack me.
Affect (How was I feeling?)
Anxious/worried/afraid.

Behavior (What did I do?)
I put my head down and walked home as fast as I could.
Consequence
Avoiding shopping mall at busy times or avoiding it completely.
Lack of food.

The response to the event is now having an impact on his functioning.
Example 2 is very similar: the person below copes with seeing faces coming
out of the wall by getting out of bed and going downstairs. The consequence
of this could be that the person becomes more and more tired, to a point
that they become sleep deprived. Lack of sleep always acts to make further
hallucinations more likely.

Example 2

Date: November 12, 2007 **Time:** 10 pm **Stress:** 75%
Event (What was happening?)
I was lying in bed last night when I started to see faces coming out of the wall.
Thought (What was I thinking?)
What is happening, am I going mad?
Affect (How was I feeling?)
Anxious/worried/afraid.
Behavior (What did I do?)
I got out of bed and went downstairs.
Consequence
The person becomes increasingly tired as their sleep pattern is disturbed due to their response to the faces.

Again, the response to the event is now having an impact on their functioning.

Symptoms

This will also offer an opportunity to look for symptoms linked to psychosis,
for example:
- In Example 1, if that pattern continued there could be a paranoia emerging.
  For further guidance read Chapter 3.
- In Example 2 again, if the pattern continued the person could be troubled
  by visual hallucinations and therefore could read Chapter 4 for further
  information.

The template is now starting to look complete and may look like Example 3 below.

Example 3

Date: November 7, 2007 **Time:** 10 pm **Stress:** 75%
Event (What was happening?)
I was lying in bed last night when I started to see faces coming out of the wall.
Thought (What was I thinking?)
What is happening, am I going mad?
Affect (How was I feeling?)
Anxious/worried/afraid.
Behavior (What did I do?)
I got out of bed and went downstairs.
Consequence
Increasingly feeling tired and becoming sleep deprived.
Symptoms
Visual hallucination – see Chapter 4.

Timelines

Another useful tool to use, both in the short and long term, is a timeline (see Figure 1.1). This is basically a chance for you to sit down with a pencil and paper and either do a long-term timeline that will chart your key life events since your first episode of psychosis, or a short-term timeline that charts key events around your last episode of psychosis.

The long-term timeline allows you to visualize what has happened since just before your first episode of psychosis to the current day. It can get you thinking about what possible key events triggered the first episode and any subsequent episodes, but also what happened to help you recover from that episode.

The short-term timeline allows you to examine more closely what happened around your last episode of psychosis. This can often be in greater detail as it will be fresher in your memory. It is useful to look at the events leading up to the episode – what you were doing, how you were feeling, and what was going on in your life at the time. Think about the events that you put on the timeline and, just as you have done with the diary template earlier, retrospectively record your thoughts, feelings, and behaviors. Think about the consequence of those events and the arising symptoms and how they affected the subsequent episode.

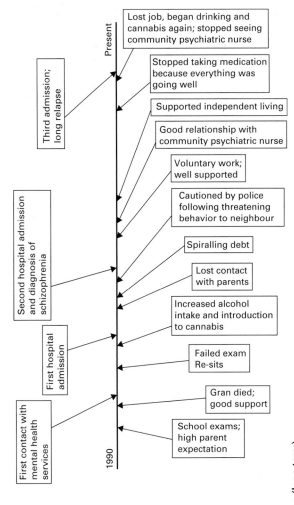

Figure 1.1 Timeline (long-term)

Case studies

Case 1

A woman, aged 24, recently diagnosed with schizophrenia following a second psychotic episode. It appeared that treatment was effective in alleviating symptoms so that from a psychosis perspective she had no problems; however, she was very upset and disturbed by her diagnosis.

Using a timeline she managed to work with her case worker and established a sequence of events that started around eight or nine months before her first episode. She had become depressed following promotion to manager of a hairdressing salon, which she had found difficult. Around this time she had started a relationship with a man that she had gradually become unsure of.

Just prior to the onset of psychosis she and her boyfriend went on holiday to Ibiza. The flight was delayed so they spent a fraught 24 hours in the airport. On arrival at Ibiza it was Halloween and her boyfriend wanted to go to a party. She was tired and wanted to go to bed, but agreed reluctantly to go with him. While there he offered to get her a drink that would "buck her up a bit." Shortly after drinking this she began to hallucinate and became very disturbed – leading to her repatriation (a very traumatic experience) and admission to hospital. Her second episode was not so dramatic, but happened a few weeks after her discharge from hospital when she went to a family wedding and became mentally unwell.

Looking at this series the woman began to see the links between the timeline and the stress vulnerability model (explained in Chapter 7). This realization was quite a cathartic experience for her.

She was terrified of the word "schizophrenia" and of reliving her psychosis. From this point she worked with her care worker developing a plan that reinforced her self-esteem and examined early warning signs and strategies for dealing with them.

Case 2

A man, in his mid 40s, with a long (20 year +) history of psychosis. Currently living in a rehabilitation hostel, Mike's history was one of multiple admissions or prison terms. He used law breaking as a means to get help, but would not admit to experiencing voices and paranoia. He was on a probation order.

The hostel staff were keen to look at ways of working with Mike, as two days earlier Mike had been aggressive and had drunk heavily leading to them not taking him on an outing. Mike was annoyed! On seeing him we agreed to examine these events, as they would get in the way of any other type of session we could have done. Using a modified timeline we looked at the events – it appeared that two days ago it was Mike's turn to cook for the hostel. He did not like doing this, as he felt that he was a bad cook. However, the cooking process included shopping for the meal, budgeting, preparation, cooking, and clearing up. This level of activity was generally alien to him and he had no confidence in his ability to do this. When shopping, he also felt that people were looking at him. As he got more uptight his voices came on, telling him how useless he was. This was the first time he had ever admitted to hearing voices. He got more anxious, the voices worsened, and he started drinking as this was his usual coping strategy for voices – "drink 'til I fall asleep."

We examined this flow of events and formulated his responses. We considered whether his responses were rational. We also considered the consequences and how they now made him feel. This allowed us to work on themes such as "are you a bad cook?" (e.g., using evidence for and against). We also looked at what other coping strategies for voices there are (e.g., distraction of a non-alcoholic nature, see Chapter 4).

Additional information. This chap also progressed in other areas (i.e., medication management and schema change).[1] He realized that he was more capable, and a better cook, than he had believed.

Case 3

Ali is a 30-year-old man with a ten-year history of schizophrenia. He lived in a hostel and was generally stable except for some aspects of negative symptoms and some residual voices ("mafia"), which he had learned to live with. He wanted to visit his parents in Dubai but was not considered well enough. He explained he had almost daily periods of going "haywire" – describing increased hallucinations, palpitations, sweating, and nausea. These occurred around 6 pm. Using a combination of a timeline and diary-keeping we established what generally happened on the days when he went "haywire" and what happened on the days he did not.

When they did occur his routine was to stay in bed until around 1 pm, get up, have a quick coffee, and then go dog walking at the local kennels.

---

[1] The term "schema" refers to an individual's thought process that leads to the formulation of a belief.

Case 3 (Continued)

He would get back to the hostel around 4.30 pm, with the main meal scheduled for 5.30 pm. On days they did not occur he would get up around 11 am, have a coffee, then go to the day center. There he would chat to friends, play cards, and have lunch, returning to the hostel around 4.30 pm. We discussed what he felt the main difference was between the two types of day, and he felt the difference was lunch, which fitted in with the aspects of his "haywire" episodes and offered a possible explanation (hypoglycaemia, i.e., low blood sugar). We could then formulate a plan that had him either eating lunch or at least having a bar of chocolate midday for two weeks. During this time he had no periods of going "haywire" at all and established a more regular pattern of getting up, which enabled him to move forward with his negative symptoms.

What was most interesting was that he identified these "haywire" periods as a problem. The professionals hardly acknowledged them, as he tended to go to bed and eat his tea later.

NB: nine months later he went to see his parents.

Cultural and religious aspects

Cultural and religious beliefs often influence the way we perceive stress and cope with it. This can make one feel that "others will not understand my perspective as I am different." It is normal to feel this way, but also important to understand that every individual is unique in this sense. As already stated in this chapter, our experiences from our formative years have a role to play. Therefore, whatever our background, a diary is a good starting point. Following the same route will make it clear that it does not matter who we are or what our experiences, ultimately the aim is to identify the problem and the stressor and learn to cope with it.

Summary

1. Keep a simple diary to help you decide where to begin.
2. Work out short timelines for problem areas.
3. Begin to share your findings with a mental health professional, carer, or friend.
4. Do not stop your medication while you work to make sense of things.

What is normal?

David Kingdon

Overview

This chapter is an antidote to stigma. Psychiatry for many years has focused on diagnosing certain mental illnesses. But what is normality? Professor Kingdon explains that psychotic symptoms can occur in anybody and that usually they clear up quickly.

Chapter contents

- Personal example
- Normal thoughts and beliefs
- Voices in the normal population
- Paranoia in the normal population
- Achieving things
- Cultural and religious aspects
- So what is normal?

Personal example

Getting up at 5 in the morning to catch a train for a 150-mile journey to Lincoln from Southampton to give a 45-minute talk and returning the same day is not normal, but it is not psychotic either. Going to Toronto from England by accident (a month early) is not clever or normal. It is mildly distressing – to me, although hilarious to my friends and family – but again not a sign of a mental health problem. So when are behaviors, thoughts, or experiences "abnormal?" It matters because if it is decided that our behavior is abnormal, we may need help – or get it whether we feel we need it or not.

"Normality" can mean, not average, extreme or failing to meet some code of behavior set by society. It can be something that is distressing or disabling, or potentially distressing or disabling, e.g., believing you can fly unassisted from the top of the Eiffel Tower and taking steps to do so, or thinking that you can save the "Free World" by invading a foreign country. Deciding what is normal is intertwined with the beliefs and customs of the culture in which you exist. If you have been elected democratically to be president or prime minister, what may seem crazy to many people may nevertheless be justified by the political system in place. Some behavior, e.g., trying to fly from heights unaided, is unlikely to be normal in any culture, but belief in spirits or alien beings varies within cultures and religions, e.g., Scientologists believe they are descended from creatures from other worlds. Is that normal? Well, in the sense we use it here, it is – because it is shared by more than the individual. Rarely, sharing of beliefs that we would call abnormal with a partner or a family member occurs, constituting a mental health problem.

Is it normal to feel despair? Not usually, but it may be considered so, if it is explained by the death of someone very close to you. It can then be seen as the inevitable cost of having had such a close relationship with all the benefits that it brought. This then creates the inevitable sense of loss when the relationship is not there. If the person wants help in coping with the loss by talking it through – with friends, family, or professionals – or even brief use of medication, that would still generally be considered "normal." It is only when recovery is not occurring – not necessarily a full return to the previous self, as that may not be possible – that we begin to consider this to be a problem with mental health. When the despair continues or the interference with the person's day-to-day life stops them doing their job, seeing people, looking after themselves, and so on, that is when some sort of intervention may be appropriate.

The difficulty can be that those around the person may think that the person needs help, when the person doesn't. Sometimes these others are being over-fussy, but often they can see that the person is distressed, or not coping, and want to help. Occasionally others are being or may be affected. It may be that the ill person doesn't think anyone can help, which is common with depression generally, but it may be that they don't know about the sort of help (not just drugs – although they may be useful) that is available. They may be embarrassed to ask, or fear the stigma that may result from seeing someone about a mental health problem. Sometimes the belief or experience the ill person has can be difficult for others to understand and be disturbing, frightening, or distressing to them. However, far from seeing it as a mental health issue they may feel direct action is to be avoided – e.g., advising not disclosing the problems to the primary care team or voluntary sector.

Normal thoughts and beliefs

What are normal thoughts and beliefs? We have a stream of thoughts going through our minds probably all the time – automatic thoughts. For much of the time they are just reflecting things happening to us or wishes, desires, or impulses that we have (see Figure 2.1).

An individual's thoughts are affected by how we feel and what happens to us, so these thoughts can become more negative if we become depressed or worried. For example, if someone close to us dies, our thoughts will inevitably be affected by this – as in Figure 2.2. These thoughts can be sad and upset at the loss but also, as time progresses, gradually move on – not necessarily forgetting what has happened but coming to terms with it. They can, however, take other forms as well – "why me?" This may be quite normal and after initially feeling angry at loss, again moving onwards usually happens, or there may be a fear of not being able to cope with the loss of the person. They may have been a source of vital support and lacking that support may make it difficult to progress.

Sometimes these sorts of rather more negative thoughts can persist and lead to someone becoming depressed in the longer term and needing help – they become abnormal. The stream of thoughts can take other courses resulting in anger towards others, e.g., doctors or nurses, or, as in the example in Figure 2.3, neighbors. To other people, these reactions can be difficult to understand – they may seem abnormal, even paranoid – but there is usually

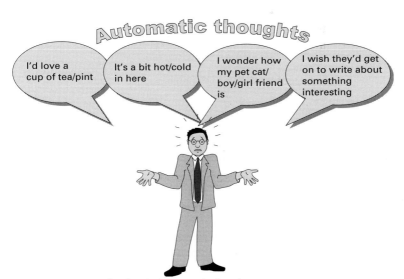

Figure 2.1 An example of typical automatic thoughts

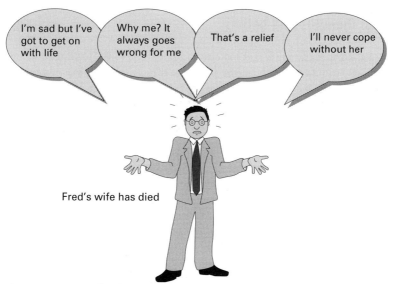

Figure 2.2 An example of sad automatic thoughts during grief

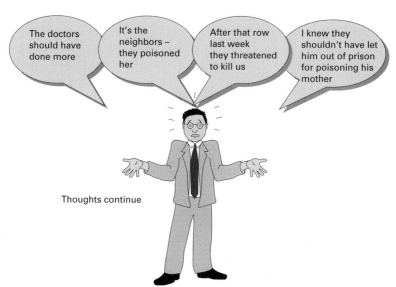

Figure 2.3 An example of paranoid automatic thoughts during grief

some reason for these thoughts developing. The example given in Figure 2.3 is a bit extreme, but possible – what is important though is that where such concerns exist, they are taken seriously and explored. Often the beliefs seem to make sense – which doesn't mean that they are right – and the reasons to

Table 2.1 Examples of normal automatic thoughts and impulses

Impulse	to hurt or harm someone
Thought	what is the calorie content of that food?
Impulse	to jump on to rails, when a tube train is approaching
Thought	of intense anger towards someone, related to a past experience
Thought	of an accident occurring to a loved one
Impulse	to say something nasty and damning to someone
Thought	of harm to, or death of, a close friend or family member
Thought	of acts of violence and sex
Thought	that something is wrong with her health
Impulse	to physically and verbally attack someone
	(Rachman & de Silva, 1978 with permission)

support them, or not, can be weighed up. In the example in Figure 2.3, although it may be understandable for Fred to believe that the neighbor was involved in his wife's death, he'd need a lot more evidence before concluding that he was – and especially for the police to believe so.

Thoughts don't need much stimulus to appear in people's minds and while most of the time they are pretty mundane, they can be very strange, violent, or sexual. Some psychologists in the 1970s got students to list all the thoughts and impulses they got over a period of time and confirmed just how odd our thoughts can be. There is a list in Table 2.1 of some of the more extreme thoughts that occurred in this group of normal people – and it has been confirmed since that these sorts of thoughts do occur quite commonly without leading to mental health problems or danger to the person themselves or others.

Thinking these thoughts can still be upsetting, but most people brush them off and move on to think about more pleasant or happier things. This certainly does not mean that the person will act on them, even though impulses can seem quite strong and even overwhelming at times. Sometimes these can become as if hypnotized or controlled in some way, but there is no evidence that, even when someone is hypnotized, they can be made to do something that is against their will. Thinking something unpleasant also doesn't say anything about the person who thinks these things – it doesn't mean they are bad, evil, or immoral. These thoughts, though unpleasant or strange in themselves, don't mean much – though they do tend to be more frequent when someone is stressed or depressed. The thoughts can also sometimes seem so vivid that it is possible the ill person will fear that others may know what these thoughts are – by some form of telepathy, for example. Fortunately, as none of us would want our innermost private thoughts made known to other people – let alone, the world – there is absolutely no evidence that this can happen. The only way people can know your thoughts is if you

Table 2.2 Beliefs in "unscientific phenomena"

68%	God
>50%	Thought transference (telepathy)
>50%	Predicting future events
>25%	Ghosts
25%	Superstitions
25%	Reincarnation
23%	Horoscopes
21%	The devil
	(Cox & Cowling, 1989)

tell them what they are. They may be able to work out that you're a bit anxious or troubled from your expression or other non-verbal communication, but they cannot read your thoughts.

Sometimes beliefs that are quite common in society (see Table 2.2), e.g., in telepathy or fortune-telling, can become overly personal. Lots of people read horoscopes but most don't rely too much on them – many people believe that some form of telepathy is possible, but not to the extent that individual messages providing personal thoughts can be transmitted. There have been scientific experiments designed to see whether telepathy is possible and the results suggest that it is not, and certainly that messages – statements like "you're no good" – cannot be transmitted telepathically.

Spiritual beliefs are very important, and to many people they can be very supportive. Faith communities provide a source of comfort and support to many going through difficulties in their lives. Occasionally thoughts or beliefs can arise that cause distress and seem related to spiritual belief, e.g., believing that the devil is speaking, usually very negatively, to you. Where the person has a strong religious belief, the spiritual leaders in their community can be very helpful in clarifying what is compatible with the person's faith and where it seems to diverge. With support, this can help them clarify the nature of their experience.

In general terms, searching for meaning when thoughts or beliefs are confusing is natural and necessary. Sometimes, though, it can lead to incorrect conclusions about individual experiences and other people's intentions, e.g., normal feelings of anxiety – upset stomach, dizziness – can be misinterpreted as being poisoned or interfered with in some way. Alternative explanations may exist to explain situations and feelings – it is very easy to jump to conclusions without taking into account all the relevant information. And once you have decided on an explanation, it can be difficult to change – in fact, we all tend to notice things that confirm what we believe and ignore the things that don't. It can be difficult to believe that something is coincidental when it seems to fit a pattern and be meaningful. It can be very hard to change your opinion – but it can and does happen. Strong beliefs, in particular, take time to change – dramatic, rapid change is unusual. Religious conversion is an example where this can happen and can be transforming, although even then there are sometimes signs that the person is getting ready over a period of time to make such a reversal of belief and can, of course, change back. When we want something badly, e.g., a relationship with some particular person, it is also possible to put one and one together and get love! However, signs can sometimes be misleading – reading desired things into a situation. Speech and even attempts to stop a person making contact, e.g., through court action, can still be read as meaning the person cares, especially where residual feelings from a past relationship exist and are misread. Non-verbal communication, e.g., the tone of our voice or way we move towards or away from someone, is very important to us in expressing emotions, but can be very imprecise and can easily be misinterpreted. Someone can look angry and because you are feeling under-confident you can wrongly think it's to do with you – when it can easily be something to do with their life, e.g., they've just been fired from their job.

Voices in the normal population

If you ask someone whether they have heard someone speaking when nobody was there, i.e., heard "voices", in the last month, about one out of every twenty-five people or so (4%) are likely to say they have. However, if you ask them if they've ever had such an experience, many more are likely to say they have. I can remember as a teenager hearing my mother's voice clearly shouting my name one evening while watching the television – only she wasn't in the room. Commonly this can happen as you are dropping off or waking up from sleep – which may be why it happened to me at that time. Hearing voices is often like "dreaming awake." It can also occur when you haven't had enough sleep – especially if this has occurred for a few nights – or when you are under other stresses. Exceptional stresses, such as being taken hostage or intense hot or cold temperature in a desert or up a mountain, can do the same. Drugs, of course, also can – and in fact we call one group, which includes speed (amphetamines), LSD, ecstasy, and cannabis, hallucinogens for this very reason. Physical illness, causing high fever for example, can also cause the same result. Generally when these things happen – and then go away – we recognize what the cause has been and just shake it off, forget it, and move on. However, when it can't be shaken off and persists, causing distress, then it begins to become abnormal.

In the 1980s, a psychiatrist called Marius Romme was intrigued by one of his patients who had developed an explanation of her voices based on a book

Table 2.3 Explanations of "voices"

- Psychodynamic: "trauma repressed"
- Jungian: "impulses from unconscious speaking"
- Mystical: "part of mind expansion"
- Spiritual: God or devil
- Parapsychological: "special gift or sensitivity, expanded consciousness, aliens, astrological"
- Medical: "chemical imbalance, schizophrenia"
- Technological explanations: satellites, etc.

(Based on Romme & Escher, 1989)

---

called *The Bicameral Mind* by Jaynes (1976). He and she went on a Dutch television program and asked people who also heard voices to get in touch. The response was much greater than they expected and around a thousand people contacted them. A conference was held where they got together and found out more about each other. About half had been in contact with mental health services but the other half had not. Some valued their experiences highly, others found them distressing. Further research has shown that many people who hear voices have mixed, positive and negative experiences – half of those with negative experiences also still have occasions when the voices can be positive. The group had a range of explanations for their experiences (see Table 2.3, which we have supplemented with further explanations that have since emerged). These explanations probably came from their spiritual and cultural beliefs and also their individual experiences. They can also reflect mood – when the person is feeling happier, voices are quieter and what they say can be pleasanter. When distressed, they can be more disturbing. In turn, unpleasant voices can cause distress and a negative cycle builds up.

So, is hearing voices normal? In a society where hearing voices is valued, it may be – from evangelical Christianity to Shamanism. Where people are under severe or certain types of stress, hearing voices may be part of a normal response. However, where they are not seen as "normal" and beliefs about them develop that are distressing to themselves or others, they are then becoming a problem, i.e., they go past being normal. It is at this point that the person may want help in coping with them, and sometimes simply to get rid of them. Sometimes the things the voices say may be frightening, disturbing, and commanding – telling you to do things, generally things that the person does not want to do. This may be to harm themselves or other people and can be very disturbing. This may be sufficient reason for others to intervene to help them avoid acting in these ways.

Paranoia in the normal population

If you ask someone if they've experienced paranoia recently, quite a lot (10–15%) will say that they have, and again many more will have had that experience at some time or another. It will depend quite a lot on their current and past experiences. If you live in a totalitarian regime, paranoia is a way of life and may be a reasonable survival strategy – being suspicious that others may be spying on you, or may report your activities to the police, was very common in the Soviet Union prior to the changes that came with glasnost. If you live in some inner city areas of England, it may be equally important to keep your wits about you, and a degree of paranoia again may be fully understandable. So, if it is quite common, when does it stop being normal? In terms of being *distressing*, it's reasonable to argue that paranoia in the inner cities or totalitarian regimes is abnormal whoever is affected by it. However, the solution wouldn't usually be to seek assistance from mental health services (and where this has happened, again in the Soviet Union in the past, such services have sometimes been used to reinforce state views of mental disorder as being any dissent against the state). Generally it is political solutions that have been more appropriate. However, it is not always as relatively straightforward as this – sometimes people in democracies, e.g., the UK and the USA, particularly when they are from minority groups, feel and may be persecuted and stigmatized. It can sometimes then be very difficult to decide when that fear of others, especially the government or police, is justified, i.e., normal, and when it is not.

Distressing paranoia can be difficult to see as normal, particularly where there doesn't seem to be a reason for it. However, the observer may not recognize the need for vigilance, e.g., if they are from a different group in society, or do not have relevant information, and the person experiencing the paranoia may have difficulty communicating it or feel that the other person is not fully trustworthy and may even be part of the problem. So, deciding what's normal can be pretty tricky.

Paranoia as an extension of social anxiety – fear of being with people – becomes a fear of them and what they might do to you. When are you paranoid and when is someone really out to get you? Is that feeling you get when you walk into a pub and it suddenly goes quiet because they were all talking about you, or just coincidence? Trauma can lead to continuing effects, for example the ongoing feeling of a need to protect oneself. Bullying can induce paranoia as a protective function.

If we think of whether paranoia is normal in terms of being "average" – happens to lots of people – then the figures given suggest it is normal. But of course the degree of paranoia and the way of responding to it, e.g., never going out of the house, can mean an abnormal reaction. But then it does seem to depend on distress or at least disabling effect – so maybe sticking to this as the key issue makes sense. But sometimes experiencing distress is seen as a price to pay for other reasons, e.g., not having to take medication, or getting financial or personal rewards that outweigh the distress.

It is important because not being normal is the lay definition of psychosis, e.g., a behaviour that is strange, bizarre, or extreme but can also be angry. Normal is established by cultural values but ultimately needs to be self-defined – except where other people are affected by an individual's behavior.

Achieving things

When we are stressed, it is normal to feel tired and want to avoid stressful circumstances, including being with casual friends, acquaintances, and strangers. Usually close friends and family can be supportive, but even then sometimes they can also be "too much trouble." Depression and negativity can then lead to avoidance of work, study, and friends. In the short term this may be inevitable and even beneficial, allowing someone to gradually rethink what has been happening to them, maybe concentrate on solving the problems they have got, or simply recover with the peace and quiet. However, for most people, it is normal to gradually begin, at their own pace, to get back to the level of contact and activity that they feel comfortable with. When this doesn't happen, it can lead to more depression and interfere with functioning so that they aren't able to do things, such as work and see friends, that they would ideally like to do. Conversely, the normal reaction of people around them can range from trying to motivate the person with gentle encouragement to the other extreme, a "get off your backside and do some work" attitude, which may be done to try to motivate but very rarely achieves that end. These "negative symptoms" in the ill person are therefore quite understandable – people need time to recover from distressing experiences, as can occur with hospitalization and with other psychological trauma – avoiding stress can reduce some of the symptoms that cause distress, such as hearing critical voices or others talking about them. Staying up at night to avoid the hectic times of the day may be part of this. In the end, return to a normal life tends to be gradual and not pressured, but with the person themselves making progress as they feel able with encouragement and sometimes guidance to do so.

Cultural and religious aspects

A lot has already been written in this chapter about religious and cultural aspects of "what is normal." Automatic thoughts are a part of life and often cultural and religious beliefs can shape these thoughts. For example, Fred who lost his wife (in Figures 2.2 and 2.3) could have grown up in a culture where it is normal to believe in "paying for sins" or "ghosts." The automatic thoughts could then become "It is my fault – I had to pay for my actions" or "She has joined the ancestral ghosts and will guide me." Similarly, the voices could be attributed to "spirits," the "devil," or "God."

Some paranoia can also be explained as normal, if one is from a different culture and experiences have not been favorable. The automatic question that can come to mind is "Is he looking at me like that because of the color of my skin?" or another example is "He did not give me the job because of my background." These thoughts may very well be based on facts, but when they begin to affect our day-to-day lives and take over our thinking they are distressing.

So what is normal?

Normality tends not to be distressing – although it can be sometimes. But if it is, this state doesn't usually go on for too long. As long as beliefs don't interfere with others, in the end it is hard to see why someone shouldn't hold them – although in the short term if one is distressed and disabled or endangered by them, other people may want to understand those beliefs and sometimes try to find acceptable alternatives to them. Normality does tend to involve agreement with others at least within your own culture about the meaning behind particular events, but some individual beliefs can still be uniquely different.

REFERENCES

Cox, D. & Cowling, P. (1989). *Are You Normal?* London: Tower Press.
Jaynes, J. (1976). *The Origin of Consciousness in the Breakdown of the Bicameral Mind.* Boston: Houghton Mifflin.
Rachman, S. J. & de Silva, P. (1978). Abnormal and normal obsessions. *Behavior Research and Therapy*, **16**, 233–48.
Romme, M. A. & Escher, A. D. M. A. C. (1989). Hearing voices. *Schizophrenia Bulletin*, **15**, 209–16.

Understanding paranoia and unusual beliefs

Paul Cromarty and Robert Dudley

Overview

This chapter aims to build on the previous chapters by giving a fuller review of paranoia and other delusions. Cognitive behavioral therapy techniques to better understand paranoia are described along with homework exercises to reduce the distress and isolation suffered by the person with excessive paranoia.

Chapter contents

- What is paranoia?
- Paranoia as a normal experience
- How common is paranoid thinking?
- Paranoia can be useful
- The down side to paranoia
- Making sense of paranoia
- Phobia examples
- Is paranoia really so odd?
- Strong fixed beliefs (delusions)
- Are you suffering from paranoia?
- Paranoia and mental illness
- Causes of paranoia
- Biochemistry
- Stress
- Alternative understanding
- Helping yourself
- Medication
- CBT for paranoia

- Putting it into action
- Building your self-esteem
- Cultural and religious aspects
- Summary

What is paranoia?

Paranoia is a term used to describe suspiciousness or mistrust. When used by people working in mental health services, it is used to describe an unrealistic or exaggerated distrust of others. This paranoia can be to the extent that other people think that there is no basis to the concerns and may consider that the paranoid person has "lost touch" with reality. Definitions of paranoia tend to be from the observer's viewpoint, as the person experiencing it often doesn't share this view at the time. Paranoia can lead to you constantly questioning or being suspicious of the motives of those people around you, and believing that certain individuals, or people in general, are "out to get me."

Paranoid ideas and behavior can occur in all of us, and also in a number of mental health problems including anxiety and depression. However, paranoia is most commonly associated with conditions such as paranoid schizophrenia, or delusional disorder.

Paranoia as a normal experience

While paranoia is common in some emotional problems, many of us have felt worried about what others think of us and their intentions towards us at some point. This can be a brief experience, such as when catching the bus late at night, walking down a dark alleyway or entering a crowded room. At these times you may be more aware of who is around, and whether you can hear people behind you. Think of the last time you walked past a group of teenagers: you may remember what it was like to be on guard and a touch paranoid. In these instances such thoughts make sense, as they have a protective function. Alternatively, these concerns can be more elaborated and longer lasting. For example, shortly after the tragic events of 9/11 or 7/7 many people reported feeling anxious owing to having a strong sense of threat and feeling unsure about what might happen next.

Personal examples

Robert

At a personal level I recall after 9/11 being in my house listening to the radio, which reported a story that crop-dusting planes in the USA had been grounded to prevent terrorists spraying poisonous gases over cities. Of course, what happened next was that I heard a light aircraft flying repeatedly over our house. We very rarely have aircraft fly overhead as we live in the city center and it seemed even more unusual that it was flying back and forth. I became anxious, and became concerned that this might be a risk to my family and me. I was concerned that this plane might be spraying poisonous gas. I went and looked up at the plane and then closed all the windows in the house. My partner was out and I was looking after my young children at the time and had not been sleeping well because of it. I convinced myself that it was all OK, primarily because the wind was blowing strongly so any poison would be dispersed in the wind.

Paul

On 9/11 I was actually in an airport in the USA about to step on to a plane. Looking back, this was just scary not paranoid; so I will describe a different experience that shows you can get paranoia without any real traumatic or threatening circumstances. Waking up with a bad hang-over one morning I decided to go for a walk for some fresh air. On passing a field of cows I suddenly noticed they were all staring at me at once. I became self-conscious and even suspicious. What were they looking at me like that for? What were they planning and why were they all looking at me in that way? I started acting as if the cows had unpleasant intentions towards me. I was thinking that the cows were having cunning thoughts and had minds. To me they appeared to be plotting and working together as if they all knew something that I didn't. I walked on but kept glancing back ... the cows continued to stare at me.

From this example we can begin to see some of the important elements for understanding paranoia and worries about other people.

Common features of suspicion and paranoia

1. Many people have these experiences.
2. They often occur in specific situations such as when we feel the need to keep ourselves safe (e.g., alone late at night).
3. These concerns may be more likely when we feel threatened or generally more anxious.
4. They may be more likely when we are stressed, not sleeping well, or not able to think clearly through drink or drugs, or a combination of all these things.
5. They are characterized by us becoming convinced that someone else is intent on harming us imminently.
6. We do not always have the chance to check out our concerns with someone else who may have helped see things in a more balanced way.
7. We take extra steps to try and keep ourselves safe, we listen out for people behind us, we check regularly for danger.
8. We do not risk finding out if we are wrong, rather we convince ourselves that we have kept ourselves safe. **Robert:** "I now believe that there was no poison on the plane, but at the time I was just relieved, my family and I were safe." **Paul:** "I am still not convinced about those cows? Hey you had to be there!"

How common is paranoid thinking?

It is all well and good saying that many people have paranoid beliefs and experiences, but what does research evidence tell us? Daniel Freeman, a psychologist at the Institute of Psychiatry in London, and his colleagues asked over 1200 students via the internet about suspiciousness and paranoia. Over a third of the participants had experienced worries about the intentions of others within the last week. The survey revealed thoughts that friends, acquaintances, or strangers might be hostile or deliberately watching them. Hence, it appears to be an everyday occurrence for many people. In fact, 52% endorsed the idea that "I need to be on my guard against others" as occurring on a weekly basis. To a lesser extent people believed that there may be someone plotting against them or there was an active conspiracy against them (8% in the last week). However, this type of study shows how common a range of paranoid thoughts can be. Similar work by Lynn Ellett and colleagues in Exeter indicated that paranoia was a common human experience, with just less than half of the participants reporting an experience of paranoia that included a clear intention of harm. So it seems possible, even quite common, for anyone to have fleeting paranoid ideas that aren't necessarily a sign of more severe mental health problems.

It is clear then that paranoid thinking is common but not everyone becomes distressed or disabled by their beliefs. It seems that within the general population between 4 and 10% of people seem to have strong beliefs including paranoid ideas that would be considered to be delusional (out of touch with reality) if interviewed by a psychiatrist. These figures are quite similar to the number of people with depression or anxiety in the general population. This is important to know as it was always assumed that paranoid ideas were rare, and hence a sign that someone was suffering from a mental illness. However, increasingly we recognize that such beliefs and ideas are relatively common and exist on a wide range of anxieties and concerns, spanning from mild suspicion to extreme fears of, and being absolutely convinced of, other people's harmful intentions towards us.

Paranoia can be useful

We can see that feeling paranoid is a relatively common experience. However, we have to ask ourselves why this might be, as no one would want to feel anxious, worried, and paranoid. While feeling paranoid or persecuted is not a pleasant experience it would seem to be true that there can be value to paranoia. In the example of walking home late at night we may feel at risk and hence check over our shoulder and prepare ourselves to be more ready to fight or seek flight (run away). As a species, humans have faced situations of genuine threat in the past and our bodies have needed to react effectively to this and to adapt. This can be traced right back to our origins with our early ancestors facing threat from other species with bigger claws and teeth, then later from our own species with improved weapons and armor. In addition, as people, we can need to be competitive and fight for resources. If you were successful, it would make sense to be concerned about other people's intentions toward you if you wished to retain your social status.

So paranoia can be useful in helping us in threatening situations (such as walking home late at night) or more long term in helping us retain our position of authority. If you look at examples from history, such as the Roman emperors or Mafia dons, you quickly see how many were murdered or betrayed by those closest to them. So to survive at the top you probably do have to assume that others are out to get you, and that trust may be foolish or even dangerous. Recently, a psychologist called Anthony Morrison, from Manchester, and his colleagues have found that people without recognized mental health problems often value paranoid/suspicious thinking, believing that paranoia helps keep a person safe. So we can see that people value using paranoia as a survival strategy.

The down side to paranoia

Of course, it may help you in some ways to be on your guard and suspicious of other's intentions. If you mistrust everyone you may think it is less likely that you will be harmed. The trouble is that many people are trustworthy, and if you adopt this view how are you going to find out? This is the problem with paranoia and mistrust. Looking out for danger all the time leaves us feeling threatened all of the time. If you feel threatened all of the time you never feel safe! It stops you from learning many situations are safe and that you can relax a lot more in them. Perhaps you could consider for yourself whether there are any advantages to feeling paranoid, and any problems or disadvantages of feeling this way.

What have been the consequences for you of feeling paranoid? Can you identify any advantages to feeling paranoid?

1.

2.

3.

What have been the consequences for you of feeling paranoid? Can you identify any disadvantages to feeling paranoid?

1.

2.

3.

Making sense of paranoia

All of this tells us that it is normal, and even useful, to feel paranoid at times. However, for most people it does not become too distressing and disrupting to their lives. When paranoia goes overboard, like a switch that we can't turn off, people may begin to lose their ability to distinguish between what's safe and what isn't. Hence, we have to understand what leads to paranoia persisting.

In recent years there have been efforts to try to understand issues such as paranoia from a psychological perspective rather than a psychiatric one. The difference here is that psychiatric illness models tend to regard problems such as paranoia as being very different to normal experiences, whereas in a psychological approach we tend to emphasize the similarities with normal experience. A psychological approach considers low mood and anxiety as being simply exaggerated normal feelings that anyone can experience. The result of this exaggeration may appear very strange and illogical at first glance to someone else, despite being understandable at a closer look. Phobias are a good example of this. Some people feel scared and threatened by situations that others are not scared of, perhaps being afraid of heights, or animals such as birds, dogs, snakes, or insects. People who are afraid of these things have thoughts that something will go wrong, they will be harmed, or at best feel stupid or embarrassed by their fears. They feel extremely distressed by these fears. They may jump to strong conclusions about the thing they fear, and often they do not wait around to see if these are true. These beliefs seem very realistic to the person having them. Others may consider it an irrational fear, as they are not afraid of spiders, wasps, or heights etc. People with the phobia often cannot understand how the thing that scares them does not bother others!

Looking at phobic anxiety is perhaps a very good way of beginning to understand paranoia as well. Both seem to be about feeling threatened and maybe feeling unable to cope with the threat itself. They both involve escaping or avoiding situations seen as threatening. They also involve constant checking or scanning of the environment to prevent further threat creeping up on them. This scanning for threat is seen as valuable, even essential to keeping safe, but it actually leaves people feeling on edge, scared, and unable to relax. If this goes on long enough people adjust their lives and restrict themselves, especially if they are sure which situations trigger the threat and unpleasant feelings that result. They think "I am sick of feeling scared and escaping from that situation, I know it is going to happen next time so I will just avoid it completely." Even when people with phobias avoid threats they aren't necessarily safe or relaxed as they may constantly scan for future threats. This is designed to make people feel safe but only makes them worse.

Paranoia is perhaps like this too. People have strong thoughts that they are under threat; mostly this will be from other people. Just having strong thoughts that someone is trying to harm you can be very scary, even if other people consider it is not true. It can lead to people feeling very threatened, wary, and mistrusting.

Phobia examples

This comparison with phobias, we think, is important for understanding paranoia. So we will consider in a bit more detail what it is like when a person has a phobia. A person afraid of wasps may believe that wasps are dangerous, and that if the person goes out these wasps will attack him or her. The belief is that wasps will target him or her above other people. In essence, they believe these wasps have harmful intentions towards them. Because of this the person may stay indoors in the summer, or only go out dressed in grey, in the belief that wasps are only attracted to bright colors. He or she will never eat sweets or drink fizzy drinks as the sugar will attract wasps.

So we can see in this example that some people with wasp phobias believe the wasps are intent on harming them, they are afraid and take steps to prevent the harm happening. They are alert and are looking out for trouble or they avoid going out if possible and if they have to, wear clothes that will not attract attention. If people unafraid of wasps understand that people who are afraid are like this because they believe they will be attacked, then the way they feel (afraid) and act starts to make more sense.

Understanding phobias in this way can be helpful in understanding a problem like paranoia. Let us consider in more detail why we may be inclined to feel paranoid from time to time.

Is paranoia really so odd?

People who think their workmates are out to get them are labelled as mad or psychotic. People who think that wasps are out to get them are labelled as worried or neurotic. Hold on a minute here! One group is seen as out of touch with reality, the other is seen as understandable and even trivialized. Thinking that an insect with a brain the size of a speck of dust is deliberately hatching plans to get you is surely no less bizarre or paranoid than thinking humans may be out to get you.

Aaron T. Beck, who invented cognitive therapy, once said that anxiety in people involved two important things:
1. **Exaggerating or overestimating a threat**, while at the same time
2. **underestimating your abilities to cope with it.**

Phobias can be understood like this, and we would argue that paranoia could be too.

Strong fixed beliefs (delusions)

When concerns about other people's harmful intentions become very strong, or very distressing, it is considered to be a sign of a mental health problem, particularly if other people think there is no basis for concern. When this is at its strongest, beliefs become very fixed and powerful and are called delusions. The big trouble with delusions is that when you get them you don't think they are delusions; you are convinced they are facts. In the same way the person with the wasp phobia is convinced that the wasps have malicious intentions toward them (as if it were fact), a person with paranoia may be convinced other people are intent on hurting or harming them.

Are you suffering from paranoia?

Psychiatric textbooks describe delusional beliefs as very fixed and rigid faulty beliefs that other people from the same culture do not hold. What this means is that people with delusions are thought to be reasoning in a way that does not appear to make sense to other people, and evidence that other people see as being obvious is not recognized by the person with the delusional belief. Persecutory beliefs are paranoid ideas held to a delusional level. For example, believing your family members have been replaced by impostors or clones that want to hurt you may be regarded as a delusional belief, as other people would not think it very plausible or realistic. Let's be honest, most people would regard it as science fiction and might react to the absurdness and miss the amount of distress it may cause.

The main feature is that in some way there is a loss of touch with reality and, of course, that means that people don't realize they are ill and have delusions. The person believes that there is some kind of threat, and it is as scary as the real thing. So how can we tell the difference? It is extremely difficult to spot signs of an illness when you don't believe you are ill in the first place. Not knowing you are ill is not just seen in mental health problems. In a host of physical health problems a person may not know he or she is ill, and may not believe someone when they are told there is a problem. For instance, for some people with high blood pressure there are no signs that there is anything the matter. The person may report feeling fine. In these cases we may need others to let us know that we are unwell. Fortunately, with paranoia there are several signs that act as clues for you when you have a paranoid illness with delusional beliefs. We will illustrate some of these signs by considering an example of what happened to a man who developed paranoid beliefs.

Case study

Tom became concerned about people conspiring against him at work. He felt very uneasy at the time, but couldn't put his finger on what this was. One day things all seemed to come to a head and he broke down after

Case study (Continued)

accusing people of plotting against him. He did not know why they were doing this to him, as Tom was in his own words "just a normal bloke." He had worked with these people for several years and considered many of his workmates as friends. He was very upset. His boss at work got a doctor to see him. Tom was in hospital for several weeks and was prescribed medication, which helped him recover. When he came home he still had occasional paranoid beliefs about his workmates. He also had them about his neighbors and even his family. This didn't make sense to him, as his family were close and supportive. In his worse moments he would get stuck looking for reasons behind a conspiracy and would constantly ask himself "Why?" This wasn't at all helpful as thoughts about conspiracy were a part of his illness. If there was no conspiracy in the first place he was never going to find one. Thinking it over this way was just making him feel anxious and threatened, and preventing him from moving on. He was also angry that workmates no longer bothered with him.

Later, he realized that if he were paranoid then the day he broke down at work wasn't the start. He had been out of sorts for several weeks leading up to this. During this time he had actually withdrawn from conversation with his workmates. He had been keeping alert for possible threats and whispers about him every day. This just made him more on edge. Everyone he approached denied conspiring against him and appeared confused by his questions. He then recalled that a couple of workmates had called to his house to see him when he first came out of hospital. He had forgotten about this, and now he remembered he was very suspicious and unfriendly toward them. He was able to see that if they were simply calling round as concerned workmates then his behavior toward them was very likely to have put them off. Tom saw that people were not likely to approach him if they expected him to be unfriendly and even accuse them of things they knew nothing about. Another possibility we discussed was that people were scared and unsure of what to do with the issue of someone they knew being mentally unwell. It is common to find some people do not know what to say to someone who has cancer, or has had a death in the family, or has been depressed or mentally ill.

From this example we can see that, for Tom, some of the signs were as follows.
1. When he asked his friends and colleagues about their behavior they looked puzzled and said they did not know what he meant.
2. A doctor was called to see him, and this did not usually happen.
3. Tom went into hospital and was offered antipsychotic medication.

4. Tom believed that long-standing friends had changed towards him.
5. Tom was not talking to his wife about his concerns.
6. Tom did not trust his family when feeling strained, which he would normally have done.

As mentioned before, knowing whether our concerns are real or not is very difficult, and keeping a sense of perspective is very hard when we are feeling anxious. From Tom's example it was clear from a number of signs that things were not right. Perhaps any one sign could have been explained away. For instance, Tom may have said to himself that his friends appeared confused when he challenged them because that was their strategy to hide their intentions. However, when all of the signs are put together it may be harder to account for all of them, and it may be important to consider on balance whether these are signs of a problem.

For yourself are there any signs that are similar that you may have noticed? Perhaps you could consider some of the questions that follow to help you find out if you are having suspicious thoughts that others may not share.

Could I be paranoid? How can I know if what is happening to me is definitely occurring or is possibly in my mind? Try and indicate if you agree or disagree with the statements.

Experience	Your assessment		
I feel that others cannot be trusted	Yes	No	Not sure
I feel that there is a plot against me	Yes	No	Not sure
I feel that somebody wants to hurt me	Yes	No	Not sure
There are meanings in the way people look at me	Yes	No	Not sure
There are messages from the TV or newspapers meant for me	Yes	No	Not sure
People are paying me particular notice	Yes	No	Not sure
I am frustrated that others don't agree with my story	Yes	No	Not sure
People are concerned for me but tell me my thoughts don't make sense	Yes	No	Not sure
Do my beliefs and suspicions really make total sense to me?	Yes	No	Not sure

---

If you have answered yes to most of these questions then there is a chance that you are feeling quite suspicious and paranoid. From these questions you could ask yourself "how would my friend/partner/parents/ brother or sister answer these for me?" If you think someone else would have a different view about whether these things were going on, how would you make sense of this?

Also ask yourself "have I always felt this way?" If you have not, what has changed, and when did it change? Have you spoken to anyone else about these experiences? If you have not, what is holding you back? It can help to talk to someone else who you trust to find out how they see it. If you have spoken to someone else, what have they said they thought was going on? Did they see it differently to you?

If you consider that there are aspects of your ideas that do not quite add up, or that others see differently, perhaps we need to consider the possibility that you are mistaken. Of course, then we need to figure out what could be happening to make you feel so bad, if the ideas you have are not quite right.

Paranoia and mental illness

While it is clear that many of us can from time to time be very concerned about the intentions of others towards us, not everyone gets so concerned that these issues become a disorder. Just like lots of us can occasionally feel sad and low, it is not the same as a persistent state of depression. Therefore, we have to understand a little more about what leads to, and what may be maintaining, a persistent fear of others.

Causes of paranoia

Genetic or family factors

Little research has been done on the role of heredity or genetics in causing paranoia. Scientists have found that the families of people with paranoia do not have higher than normal rates of either schizophrenia or depression. Whether paranoid disorder, or a predisposition to it, is inherited is not yet known.

Biochemistry

The discovery that psychotic illness (where the person is meant to have lost touch with reality) can be improved with antipsychotic medication led researchers to look for the causes in abnormal brain chemistry. The findings are very complex, as more and more of the chemical substances that carry messages from one nerve cell to another (neurotransmitters) have been discovered. So far, no definite answers have been found. In modern psychiatry, medication is widely prescribed as an effective means to improve or control symptoms, but it is still not known whether biochemical brain changes cause paranoia.

Abuse of drugs such as amphetamines, cocaine, marijuana, LSD, or other stimulants or "psychedelic" drugs can lead to paranoia. People with major mental health problems such as paranoid schizophrenia may find that their symptoms become worse under the influence of these drugs. Cannabis is increasingly being linked to the onset and continuation of paranoia, perhaps owing to its increased strength or maybe more widespread use.

Stress

Some researchers consider that paranoia may be a reaction to high levels of life stress. Lending support to this view is evidence that paranoia is more common among immigrants, prisoners of war, and other people undergoing severe stress. Sometimes, when thrust into a new and highly stressful situation, people suffer an intense form, called "acute paranoia," in which paranoid ideas develop over a short period of time and last only a few months.

One thing we know is that persecutory beliefs can develop at a time of great difficulty and stress. For instance, if we are being bullied, or are the victims of assault or other *trauma* of one sort or another it may be the trigger for a paranoid belief. Increasingly, we are coming to understand that if bad events have happened to people growing up then this can make them more prone to mental health problems generally, and to paranoia. John Read, a psychologist based in New Zealand, has examined the types of life events experienced by people with paranoia and found that many have been bullied, or have been victims of sexual and physical assault. Hence, we can see that these distressing ideas can emerge from a time of genuine difficulty. So some traumatic events may trigger paranoia, or perhaps having a lot of unpleasant things happen to you when growing up may generally increase a person's vulnerability or risk factor for later problems.

Therefore, a vulnerability to paranoia may have developed out of genuine adversity. Similarly, people can and do face *genuine* current threats. People are victims of crime, intimidation, and threats, and strange things do happen to people. For instance, people can apparently steal your identity, and hence we must always consider that there may be some real truth to what is going on at present, or that something may have happened in the past. However, we must also consider that we may be mistaken, particularly if we are still acting as if the threat were real when in fact it is no longer present. Even if we were bullied at school, it does not mean that everyone will act the same way now we are adults. If we felt unable to cope with threats in the past, we may well feel the same in the present. If we have faced adversity in the past, we may look out for and overestimate threat, and doubt our abilities to cope with it. This may say more about our own beliefs that we carry into situations than the situations themselves, and could make us wary and mistrusting in many situations where others may not be and where there is no need to be.

The truth of the matter is we do not know what causes paranoia. It could be genetics, a brain abnormality, or early upbringing that could all predispose a person to paranoia; current stress may act as a trigger. It could be a combination of all these.

While it is helpful to understand what may have caused the problem, a psychological approach such as CBT is more concerned with treating what *maintains* the problem. Focusing on what is keeping the problem going is common when working with problems such as phobias, and has been proven to produce better outcomes and reduce symptoms far more successfully than discussing causes. Often the causes are clear, for instance someone who is afraid of dogs may have been bitten by a dog some years ago. However, once established, people do things that keep the phobia, or other problem, going and stop their beliefs changing. For example, running away or avoiding dogs, wasps, heights, snakes, people, and places may provide some short-term relief, but this does not allow you to discover that you weren't in any danger in the first place. Staying put in these situations would allow you to find out that you were in fact safe, and consequently scary thoughts and feelings would reduce.

Once a belief that you are at risk has been established, it may be kept going by reasoning processes. For instance, people with delusional beliefs have been shown to demonstrate more often a *jumping to conclusions* style of reasoning. This means that people with delusional beliefs, usually paranoid ideas, may make up their minds more hastily and readily than people without such beliefs. This is not true of everyone with paranoia, but somewhere between 40 and 70% of sufferers seem to have this style. This in itself is not too problematic; making your mind up quickly can be fine if you come to the right decision. However, when you are making your mind up about emotionally upsetting issues, then a hasty style can increase the chance of making errors.

Furthermore, we know from the work of Richard Bentall, Peter Kinderman, Sue Kaney, and others that people with paranoid beliefs have a characteristic *attributional* style. By this we mean that when something bad happens people with paranoid ideas tend to blame other people for the bad event. People with depression are more likely to blame themselves if something goes wrong, whereas people without paranoia or depression will generally blame the situation or bad luck. For instance, if you parked your car and came back to find it scratched, a depressed person would likely blame themselves for parking it in a place where this could happen. A person with paranoid ideas may consider that another person deliberately scratched their car and not others people's cars. A person with neither depression nor paranoia may just think they parked in the wrong place at the wrong time, and it was bad luck and feel angry that it had happened. Once again, there is nothing in itself bad or wrong about these different styles, but they may mean that people with paranoia may more often look to blame another person when actually it may just be bad luck, circumstances, or coincidence.

Another problem that may lead to people's suspicious ideas being maintained is a lack of consideration of *alternative* explanations. This often seems to happen as people take experiences to have significance or meaning related to themselves. Take, for example, hearing a person in a shop cough. When we are feeling very anxious and paranoid we may take this cough to have meaning. We may see the person coughing as being part of the conspiracy, and intent on hurtingus. However, we have confused the cough, which is real, with the perceived meaning ("he is intent on hurting me"), which may or may not be real. There may actually be lots of reasons why someone coughed. Also, we may hear other noises and sounds that make us suspicious. Hearing a muffled conversation from the neighbor's house may make us concerned that "they are keeping their voices low while talking about me." We may not stop to think that from their house our voices probably sound muffled to them.

A further feature of paranoid beliefs is the tendency to misinterpret *chance* events as having meaning. If we go on holiday and meet a neighbor we may ask ourselves "what is the chance of that", and consider that it is very unlikely and it must have a reason. Actually, we have all usually had this kind of experience; the problem is when we are on guard we can find meaning and relationships in things that we do not usually notice. For instance, seeing a car number plate with our initials may seem to have a meaning that it is sending us a message. Or seeing someone wearing the same coat as yourself may mean to you that the person is following you to the shops you go to, rather than the shop sells a lot of coats like yours. The main message is that chance events happen frequently, and if we are really looking for coincidences and meaning there are actually lots out there to find. Next time you are out in a car, notice how many are exactly the same make and color. It is not usually long before you see the same car as your own. The important thing to remember is that people are capable of reading things into situations that may not always be there, or that can be explained by other reasons we don't think of or consider.

Of course, people can feel paranoid because of *voices* they hear. In the chapter on hearing voices (Chapter 4) we will learn that people may be worried about what the voices say, or whose voice it is. These experiences can serve to maintain our sense of paranoia. If it is possible to reduce the frequency or impact of the voices, by using some of the approaches described in Chapter 4, then this may reduce how paranoid you feel.

As with all other emotional problems, we understand that what we do to keep ourselves *safe* can actually lead to us continuing to feel at risk and suspicious. For instance, if I never go out, in order to avoid being attacked,

I will never find out if I am still at risk. If, when I am out, I only look down at the floor to stop people recognizing me, I will never find out whether people are really looking out for me. Hence, how we try to cope can stop us finding out if things are really as risky as we fear. Moreover, to keep ourselves safe we sometimes attack the threat. So, if we are afraid of a wasp we may step on the wasp before it can attack us. Of course the wasp may never have attacked. Or worse, if the wasp is not killed, it may actually then attack. Similarly, sometimes people with paranoia may become aggressive to, or accusing of, people around them when they feel threatened, in order to keep people away. Unfortunately, this will probably just draw more notice and attention to yourself, which often is the opposite of what you want.

Some of these issues are shown in a model (see Figure 3.1). These factors are thought to be part of what may lead some people to experience paranoia, and it is based on the work of Daniel Freeman and his colleagues (Freeman, Freeman, and Garety, 2006).

Can you see if any of the factors outlined in Figure 3.1 apply to you?

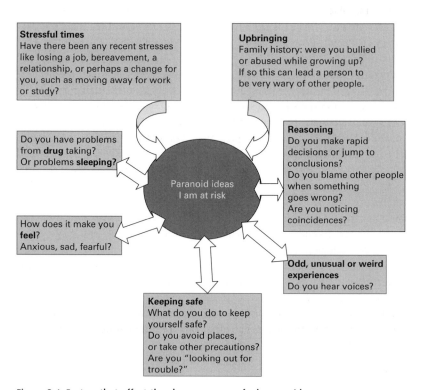

Figure 3.1 Factors that affect the chance we may feel paranoid

Alternative understanding

Perhaps we need to consider whether your problem is like a phobia. It isn't about being under threat; it is about feeling threatened when you are just as safe as usual.

Your problem isn't about conspiracy, the CIA, Mafia, government, your neighbors, workmates, aliens, terrorists, and so on. It is about your beliefs and what is inside your mind. Perhaps you have a people phobia, or a phobia of trusting people?

Helping yourself

Of course this could be wrong, your view of it could be true, and you are right to feel upset. However, perhaps we need to try and find out if there is another way of seeing it and at least consider the chance that there is another explanation.

The first place to start is to consider whether you are taking care of yourself. Are you sleeping OK? If you are not sleeping well consider whether there are steps you can take to improve this (good sleep tips are available at www.MywebLiving.com/Insomnia). This is important as poor sleep makes it much harder to cope. Similarly, if you are taking drugs, or alcohol, find out how you can reduce these perhaps by seeing your primary care physician.

Secondly, ask yourself what led to you first experiencing your worries about others? Have you been through a stressful time? Have you been the victim of bullying, real persecution, or abuse, while growing up or more recently, before the development of your concerns about other people? If you have been affected in this way then it is not surprising you would be mistrustful or concerned about others, and you may want to seek the help of a CBT therapist or clinical psychologist to help you deal with the effects of these types of experiences (the British Psychological Society website www.bps.org.uk or the British Association of Behavioural and Cognitive Psychotherapies website www.babcp.com are good places to find out more).

Have you spoken to other people about your concerns? Is there someone you feel you can trust to talk to about these ideas? Talking to someone you feel you can trust will be a big important first step. This may be a friend or member of the family. For some people it can be their family doctor. Your doctor can refer you to see a psychiatrist or other mental health worker who has more expertise in these matters. For many people this is helpful, while for others who are already mistrusting and suspicious this is scary. Some people are afraid of being put in hospital and fear that they will be labeled as mad. Others prefer to be in hospital and say they feel safe there. If you do have concerns about going to see your doctor or someone from your local mental health services there is often information about these that you can read beforehand. There are alternatives too. You can check lots of things via the internet or at local community centers or libraries. There are also voluntary agencies and charities, such as MIND, that you may feel more comfortable approaching or using as a first step.

If you have been experiencing high levels of stress it is important that efforts are made to help reduce or remove stresses by getting appropriate help. You do not have to deal with this alone as there are services available that can help with housing, money, and similar difficulties.

Medication

Have you been prescribed medication? If so are you taking it? In some, but not all, cases medication can help reduce the frequency or the distress of paranoid ideas. It may help you, and you may need to speak to a doctor about a trial of medication. Antipsychotic medication such as haloperidol, chlorpromazine, clozapine, risperidone, quetiapine, olanzapine, or aripriprazol may be prescribed by a primary care physician or psychiatrist. You can use medication as a test. What if you took it as a trial and after a few weeks your suspiciousness, fearful beliefs, and sense of threat started to go away? What might this be telling you? Further information on taking medication can be found in Chapter 6.

Cognitive behavioral therapy for paranoia

Another way to help yourself is to try and consider whether there are other possible explanations for what is going on: in essence, considering another point of view. However, we know that changing our views is difficult. A researcher called Roberts reported in 1991 that he had asked people about their paranoid beliefs, and asked whether they wanted to be proved wrong. Actually, they did not want to be proved wrong. They did not want to be shown that the FBI (for instance) were not following them, they wanted help to stop the FBI following them. What this shows us is that we may have to work very hard to consider we could be mistaken, and that it is hard to ask ourselves if we can find out if there is another viewpoint.

When trying to see if there is another point of view the first task is to try and note down your thoughts. A diary or thought record can be very helpful in this process. For example, the template below could be used to help us see when and where you tend to get these paranoid thoughts. An example of how to fill it in is included. Perhaps you could try filling it in for yourself, considering the last time you felt particularly worried about other people.

Completing your thought record

Situation	Feelings	Thoughts	Actions
Note down where you were, who with, what was going on.	What did you feel emotionally?	Write down what you were thinking to yourself.	What did you do in this situation to help manage your feelings?
I was in the newsagents and I heard a man cough.	*Frightened, paranoid.*	*He is part of them, they do not like me, and I am going to get attacked.*	*Left the shop and went home quickly.*

When you have filled in your thought record then there are some simple questions to ask yourself at the beginning.

Am I *overestimating* the level of threat? How do others see this situation? How did I used to see these situations in the past? Could it be less dangerous than I thought? A little like with the person afraid of wasps, is it possible I am seeing too much danger in this situation?

Am I *jumping to conclusions*? Are you making your mind up on the basis of very little evidence? For instance, in the example, a cough was seen as evidence of the conspiracy. Ask yourself "Am I looking for trouble or taking things to heart?" Here we can see that the person not only made up his mind quickly, but it was also seen as directly relevant to himself; he took the cough to be directed at him. It has been suggested that whenever we make up our minds we should always consider if there is more than one possibility for the event. Take an example such as going out in the morning to go to work and your car did not start. What explanations may there be? Someone has stolen the engine, the car may have a flat battery, it may be a cold morning, there may be a loose wire, or the car may be out of petrol, and so on. These may all be possible explanations.

If you decided it was a flat battery and went and bought a new one, and actually it was because the car was out of petrol, then you made a rapid judgment that cost you time and money. Hence, whenever we face a situation it is helpful if you can consider whether there is another possibility that may have caused the experience. This may help slow down your decision making, and lead you to seeking more information that may help you decide which explanation best fits the facts.

Am I *blaming* someone else for this bad event? Are there any other explanations I am missing, like it being bad luck or misfortune? This happens in life from time to time. We know from the work of Richard Bentall and others that people with paranoia have a tendency to blame people rather than circumstances for bad events. In this example this may not be relevant, but for yourself are there any other possible factors that led to the event happening? Could you blame the situation, rather than there being another person to blame?

A further strategy for considering whether there may be other possible explanations for what is going on is to consider all the other reasons for the original event. This can be difficult as we often mix up what we saw or heard happen (a cough) with the explanation for this event (it was a sign). So, what we need to do is make sure we are looking at other possible reasons for someone coughing. First of all, ask yourself how strongly you believe your explanation. Give it a rating out of 100, with 100 meaning that you believe it completely (not a shadow of doubt) and 0 being you do not believe it in the slightest. Then try and list all the possible reasons why people cough, and at the end of the list place your explanation; in the example it would be "Because it was a sign that was directed at me." Then indicate how much you believe the explanations for these other reasons could be possible by putting a percentage value on them, as shown below.

The person had a cold   35%
The person had an allergy   15%
The person was a smoker   25%

When you have done this, add your explanation, and consider how much you believe this in light of these other possibilities.

It was directed at me   25%

This can be visually represented as pieces of a pie or cake (see Figure 3.2), and can help show us all the other possible explanations that may have led to the person coughing. We do not know if any are true, but the important part is that we do not know that any of them are not true either; they are all possibilities. However, it may make you feel slightly less distressed if other possibilities may exist. If you find it hard to think of other possible explanations, it may help to ask a friend or family member who you trust what other reasons they can think of. This may help you consider some possibilities you had not thought about.

For the example that Robert described (see page 37), about the plane flying overhead, he would have needed to consider what other reasons there may be for a plane flying overhead repeatedly. It could have been a learner practicing, or a surveyor or mapping plane, or even just someone flying back and forth to look at the city. If he could have thought of these at the time, it may have made him feel less worried.

Cognitive behavioral therapy tries to help with paranoia by looking at alternative explanations to rationalize fears and predictions. However, these

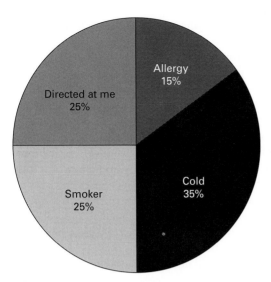

Figure 3.2 Chart showing other possible explanations for why someone may cough

are just possibilities, until we begin to try to act differently, to help find out which if any of our possibilities are most realistic. In order to really learn if we are as at risk as we fear we are, we have to try to act differently.

Putting it into action

So far we have considered other possible explanations, but at this stage they are all just possibilities, and you may still be feeling just as bad. It is time to consider putting some of these possibilities to the test. We do this in CBT with what are called behavioral experiments. We think that they are helpful in finding out about our ideas and beliefs. To overcome our fears takes great courage and the process is not easy. It can help to have someone trusted and close to you, to help you undertake some of these tasks.

It is an integral part of CBT that the upsetting thoughts are examined and checked out in some way. Behavioral experiments involve planning and undertaking an activity that helps challenge or shed new light on the thought. The primary purpose of these tasks is to help find out if your experiences are genuine or whether you may have a people phobia. One obvious benefit of behavioral experiments is that we put into action what we have talked about. You could not learn to ride a bike by talking about it; you can give it some thought but eventually you have to get out there and try.

Melanie Fennell, a psychologist from Oxford, describes how behavioral experiments will usually be undertaken following a number of steps that are similar to those involved in carrying out scientific research. These steps are:

1. *Make a prediction.* It is important to state clearly what the thought is that is being tested and to specify what will be the outcome. These are often phrased as "if ... then" statements. For instance, "if I see someone scratch their nose, then I know he has heard about me on the internet and will try and beat me up."

2. *Review existing evidence for and against the prediction.* In keeping with the previous section on considering other possible explanations, consider how likely you think it is that something will happen or not. In this case consider whether you will see someone scratch their nose and whether they may be doing this for any other reason. This may help you begin to determine if there is an alternative explanation that has not yet been considered, or one that you do not believe very much. For example "I saw someone scratch their nose when they could not have seen me watching, and did not know I was there, and I did not think he was going to hurt me. I decided that his nose was itchy and so he was scratching it." Hence an alternative explanation is that "maybe scratching your nose is normal."

3. *Devise an experiment to test the prediction.* It is important that the test is specific and has a clear outcome. For instance, "if you saw someone scratch their nose and you thought that it meant you were at risk, what would be the signs, how would we know?" These need to be specified as features that you can see (i.e., someone watching you, someone following, someone moving hostilely toward you, etc.). The experiment has to have a time frame in which it will be undertaken as well. Set a day and a time when you are going to do this. An alternative prediction needs to be specified in advance as well. For instance, "if you see someone scratch their nose and no one stares at you in a hostile way or makes faces about you, what would that show us?" If the answer is that they scratched it because they were trying to fool me then we may not discover anything new in this experiment. If the alternative prediction is not something like "scratching the nose may be normal and common," we have to ask whether the experiment can work.

4. *Perform the test and note the results.* Go out and try the test. Take someone you trust with you, and compare notes as to what you are finding out.

5. *Draw conclusions.* With your friend review or look over the results and compare the original idea and the alternative. It is important to consider whether the experience or test better supports the initial prediction or the alternative.

Here are some other examples of changing behavior that people have found helpful. A man with paranoia believed that people were laughing at him because they had heard rumours spread about him that he is gay. To cope with this and reduce the chance of people laughing he walked with his head down in order to keep a low profile. What problems do you think there might be with this strategy?

For this person one problem was that when people did laugh when he was nearby (for whatever reason) he was less likely to see the cause of the laughter. Hence, an experiment for him was just to walk with his head raised in order to see what he noticed about people laughing. He predicted that people would be laughing at him, and not for any other reason. An alternative explanation was that people laugh for lots of reasons, which may not have anything to do with him, but by keeping his head down he was missing these other possible explanations. By doing this he learned that people laugh for lots of reasons and not just to do with him.

Another example was of a man who had a paranoid belief that rumors were being spread on the internet about him. One test was to do an internet search looking for this rumor. The person predicted that if we looked it would be easy to find the site with the allegations on, as everyone knows about them. Our alternative was that he was worried about what other people thought about him, and that actually no website would be easily found. Therefore, we looked on the internet and could not find a reference to him. This made him consider the possibility that he could be mistaken.

Of course, it is not all about trying to prove yourself wrong; it is just as important to think of experiments that can build up evidence for the less distressing alternative explanation. For instance, if you think people are going to hurt you because they think you are a nasty person, then we can devise experiments to help demonstrate that you are acceptable to others and no different to anyone else. If the experiment was to ring a friend, a person with this concern may predict that the friend would react in a cold and rejecting manner (i.e., sound unhappy to hear from them, not ask them about themselves, hang up, etc.). A test of being acceptable would be the opposite of these predictions (being asked how they are, talking for more than two minutes, etc.). He may try and ring a friend he has not spoken to for a considerable length of time. Before he did we had to consider what would be the signs that his friend thought he was likeable and acceptable. There may be some signs that include tone of voice, the length of the conversation, whether the friend asked any questions about him, and any outcomes such as agreeing to speak or meet again. Note the way the experiment was set up as a test of the idea that he is acceptable and likeable. We did not go looking for signs that he was unacceptable or that his friend would reject him. Here we are using an experiment to test the alternative rather than try and prove he is wrong about the original thought. From this experiment arose a series of further experiments such as ringing other people, about whom he was less certain of their response.

The goal of all of this work is to begin to see if there is a better, less threatening, explanation of how the world and other people really are.

Perhaps they (like wasps) are not as threatening or scary as you believe. Perhaps you have a people phobia.

Coping

Sometimes it is not possible to consider whether your beliefs are right or wrong. It can be too frightening or too confusing. In these instances, sometimes it is better to build on one's strengths, and address what you can control.

Building your self-esteem

Paranoid thoughts very often feed off low self-esteem. If you believe, or fear, that you may be a bad person, or are unlovable, or are a failure or reject, then it is likely that it is easier to believe that others do not like you, or may want to hurt you. When you have been poorly for a long time it may be difficult to know how valuable you are. So ask yourself who you are and what is your worth? We should probably all ask ourselves these questions because very often we have decided in childhood that we are "a loser" or "useless" when in actual fact we are OK. Feeling good about yourself means that it is less likely that others will see the bad in you. Again these feelings of low self-esteem can affect people with phobias. They feel relieved at avoiding their feared situation, but the longer this goes on the more they feel restricted, out of control, silly, or even a failure for not being able to cope.

> Pauline Hall and Nick Tarrier from Manchester, England, reported that when people with psychosis, including paranoid beliefs, identified good qualities about themselves (for example "I am thoughtful," "I have a good sense of humour," "I am good at football," etc.) and asked people to try and increase these positive qualities, they felt much better about themselves. The people had to try and do more or improve on these positive aspects of themselves. Just doing this made them feel better generally, and reduced how bothered a person was by problems such as voices or paranoia.

What are your good qualities? List them here, being as specific as you can (i.e., not just "I am kind;" try and spell out what makes you kind – how do you act, what do you say?) then use this as the basis to try and increase the use of these good qualities.

1.

2.

3.

4.

5.

6.

Cultural and religious aspects

Case study

Sheila, of African Caribbean origin and currently residing in the UK, was going through a difficult divorce from her husband who was American. They had a son from the marriage who now lived with Sheila. It was not easy being a single mother, especially as Sheila had grown up in a large family who supported each other back home. Since arriving in the UK, she had always been very conscious about her privacy from neighbors. As the situation became more stressful, she struggled to cope with day-to-day life. Her self-consciousness and need for privacy started growing and becoming a problem. She started believing that her neighbors were watching her and were spying on her for her ex-husband. This feeling grew further and she then started believing that her neighbors were being "racist" toward her and were out to get her because of her color. She became extremely distressed and eventually locked herself and her son in the house.

From this example, it is obvious that paranoid ideas can occur irrespective of cultural background or religious beliefs. Sometimes, coming from a different cultural background can add to an individual's stresses, e.g., through isolation, lack of family and social supports, and difficulties with adjustment. Often the theme of the paranoid ideas can be culturally dictated as well. However, it is important to recognize that these symptoms are common across cultures, and can be helped. There is no shame in discussing these symptoms just because your cultural background is different.

Summary

Paranoid ideas are common, and can be very distressing. They can occur for a whole host of reasons including stress, poor sleep, drug use, and so on. When people develop these ideas it is often hard to know that we have ideas or beliefs that others do not consider reasonable or realistic, and we have to work hard to step back and consider all the possibilities. Considering your paranoia as a type of phobia may be a helpful step; it makes it feel more normal, and phobias can be treated successfully with CBT. While it is not an easy process and requires bravery and effort on your part, it is possible to improve how you feel by considering in more detail your thoughts, or building on your strengths.

FURTHER READING

Bentall, R. (2003). *Madness Explained: Psychosis and Human Nature.* Allen Lane: The Penguin Press. (This is a book about psychotic illnesses including paranoia. It covers a lot of the history and theory about paranoia and mental health problems.)

Freeman, D., Garety, P. A., Bebbington, P. E., *et al.* (2005). Psychological investigation of the structure of paranoia in a non-clinical population. *British Journal of Psychiatry,* **186**, 427–35. (This is a research report that helps us understand how very common are suspiciousness and paranoia.)

Freeman, D., Freeman, J. & Garety, P. (2006). *Overcoming Paranoid and Suspicious Thoughts.* London: Robinson. (This is a self-help book that helps develop an understanding of suspiciousness and paranoia.)

Voices

Douglas Turkington

Overview

This chapter aims to offer the reader an understanding of voice hearing and other hallucinations. The importance of engaging with the voices and developing viable coping strategies is stressed.

Normally people communicate by talking to each other. This seems like an obvious statement but what of the situation when we hear a voice talking to us when there is nobody about? This is the puzzling situation of "hallucinating." The experience of voice hearing is uncanny because the voices sound exactly like normal voices. They can be loud or quiet, and sound very clear and real. The first point to make in relation to voice hearing is that it is a normal human experience just like feeling nervous before giving a wedding speech. Every single human person in the world has probably experienced a hallucination at some point in their life. For many people it is not a voice they hear but a sound; virtually everybody has the experience at some point of awakening from a deep sleep to hear a bell ringing or someone call their name. When fully awake they realize that although it sounded very real it was not caused by anybody or anything in the room. Most people conclude that this experience was just part of waking up and think no more about it. I can give an example from my own experience.

Example 1 Hearing voices

I was wakening from a deep sleep when I was 32 years old. As I emerged from the depths of slumber I clearly heard my dad calling my name; he was shouting loudly "Douglas . . . Douglas." I quickly became awake and looked around a bit shocked by what I had heard. There was nobody there and I knew that my dad was back in Scotland and his voice sounded younger than it is now. It then came to mind that I had heard him once shout like this. I was snorkelling off the coast of Majorca and a jet ski was being driven at high speed in my direction. Just as my dad shouted I dived beneath the surface to collect a shell from the sea floor and looking up saw the jet ski pass at high speed over the area where I had been swimming.

This example from my own experience raises some important points:
1. Sleep and awakening is in some way linked to voice hearing.
2. The voice that is heard sounds completely real.
3. The voice will produce an emotional reaction (in my case shock).
4. The voice is saying something meaningful for the voice hearer.
5. The voice can refer to a stressful incident from the past, which has perhaps not been emotionally resolved or examined.
6. By working out the message being delivered by the voice there is often a need to address an emotional issue. In my case I thought about the fact that I had been nearly killed by the jet ski and spoke to my father about the incident, which was worthwhile as we had both never spoken about it.

How common is voice hearing?

Voice hearing is therefore a very common experience and one that does not usually mean mental illness. Voice hearing for most people is a transient experience that does not require medication or therapy. It is said that 10–15% of people will have a longer period of hallucinating, over days or weeks, at some point in their lives, and usually this is linked to stress. It is calculated that one person in forty has this experience each year. This is an extremely large number of people, about the same number who see a football match at some point in the year. As Marius Romme described, these voice hearers are not in contact with psychiatry and continue in their employment and relationships. Often they view the voices in a positive way, e.g., as memories from childhood, as part of their psychological development or as a special gift. The attitude that is taken to the voice hearing experience is one of the most important determinants as to whether there is a good or a poor outcome. People who cope well with episodes of voice hearing have one other characteristic. They have developed a relationship with their voices that allows them to control the experience.

Voice hearing and mental illness

Although voice hearing, like anxiety, sadness, and unusual beliefs, is normal throughout human society, each of these conditions, if very extreme or persistent, can be seen as being part of a nervous breakdown (mental illness) for which professional help might be needed. Voices in emotionally unstable personality disorder only come at times of extreme personal stress. Very sad and negative voices are often heard in psychotic depression. In schizophrenia, voices are often making unpleasant comments or telling the person to do things they don't want to do. The suggestions given in this chapter to help improve one's ability to cope with voices are meant to supplement the treatment already being given for any of the mental illnesses mentioned above. In particular, antidepressant or antipsychotic medication should never be stopped unless this has been agreed with your primary care physician or psychiatrist. Voices in many people are worsened by drugs such as cannabis, LSD, amphetamine, or ecstasy. Even when a person finds that using cannabis can make them feel relaxed, it has been found that cannabis use can make the chance of having voice experiences more likely. So even though it seems to help it may actually make things worse. Often those who experience voices due to illegal drug use also suffer from the unpleasant feeling of paranoia: "people are talking about me ... they are out to get me ... my life is at risk." Ways of dealing with such paranoid thoughts have been addressed in Chapter 3.

Example 2 Voices in schizophrenia

Norman listed the following unpleasant voices:
   "He has no friends."
   "He is a waster."

Example 2 (Continued)

"Just stay in bed."

"Why doesn't he take an overdose . . . his parents would be better off without him."

The voices were reported to be present for up to 60% of his waking hours and due to their unpleasant and critical comments he had become demoralized. The voices would often speak to each other and he would spend hours listening to their unpleasant discussion and arguments about what he should do. He had given in to the voices, and was staying in bed, although he was taking his medication. The medication definitely helped dull the voices a bit, but his quality of life as such was very poor. He needed help to understand the voices, to begin to take some control, and to initiate some coping strategies. Only then could he begin to aim for some worthwhile life goals.

Anybody in this situation really needs a community psychiatric nurse or psychologist with training in CBT to help them to make sense of their voice hearing, and to begin to take control again. Voices therefore can be a sign of a variety of different mental illnesses as well as being seen in illegal drug misuse and in the normal population.

Keeping a voice diary

The first step in relation to distressing voices is to be scientific and keep a record of how often they come on and in what situations. Once we have more knowledge about the voice hearing we can then begin to consider what the cause might be. The very act of keeping a diary can lead to surprising insights into possible ways to cope. Sherlock Holmes once said to Dr. Watson "data, data, data . . . my dear Watson . . . I can't make bricks without clay." Like Sherlock Holmes we need more information about the voices. The instructions for completing the voice diary are fairly simple – for each different situation during the day write down whether the voice is present, what it says and how loud it is. The issue of loudness is scored between 0 and 10, where 0 is an extremely quiet voice and 10 a voice that is shouting as loudly as possible.

Example 3 Use of a simple voice diary

Fiona had been a successful accountant until she took on too much work and started not to sleep well. She found herself becoming increasingly stressed and anxious. Next she began to hear whispers in the corner of the room. These gradually became louder and more nasty. Eventually, in an exhausted state, puzzled and distressed by the voices she resigned from her job and ended up being seen for home treatment by the Assertive Outreach Team. She was very embarrassed by what the voices were saying to her and she requested a female worker to help her.

These instructions were given for the voice diary.
1. For the first week just continue with your normal daily routine and each time you do something (Column 1) observe whether or not the voice is present (Column 2).
2. If the voice is speaking do not do anything in particular, just be interested in what it has to say and write a few lines about this (Column 3).
3. In Column 4 we would like a score for how loud the voice is: 10/10 is maximum loudness and 1/10 a very soft whisper.

Often people fill in the diary at the end of the day. The only problem with this is that most of the information is often forgotten. It is better to take the diary with you and fill in a few lines every now and again as you go through your day. If it is difficult to carry the diary with you then by all means complete as much as you can at the end of the day. Getting a little bit done is better than nothing at all. If the voices say things that are too embarrassing to write down then keep these things in mind to report to your nurse or psychologist when you next see them.

An example of a completed voice diary

Situation	Voice present?	What did voice say?	Loudness 1/10
Breakfast	No		
Shower	Yes	"You need to wash"	4
Reading the paper	Yes	"You are the cause of all the trouble"	3
Shopping	Yes	"Don't try to hide, they all know about her . . . she's a slut"	9
Relaxation class	yes	"She will be punished for this"	6
Listening to classical music	Yes	"She needs new clothes"	1
Cooking dinner	No		

Voice diary template

Situation	Voice present?	What did voice say?	Loudness 1/10
Insert your own daily activities below.	Is the voice talking during this activity? Yes or no.	Write down the exact words used if possible (no matter how unpleasant or strange).	Enter the voice score out of 10 for loudness.

Working with a voice diary

Hopefully you will now have a record in your diary of a day of voice hearing. Let's first look at the example given. What do you notice? Firstly the voice is not present all day long. It would seem that during sleep, breakfast, and when cooking dinner the voices were not active. Also there seemed to be certain activities that were liable to cause an increase in the loudness of the voice. The diary seemed to show that listening to classical music, at least on the day in question, led to a very low level of voice activity. Did your voices vary in a similar way? It looks like for Fiona cooking and classical music could be good coping strategies. Did anything in your diary seem to be related to low levels of voices? If so, then make a note of this here.

Possible coping strategies:

1.

2.

When, during the day, were Fiona's voices loudest and most upsetting? From the diary we see that they were loudest when she was out shopping and when in the relaxation class. How do we explain this? Do you have any specific times when the voices are louder? If so, please note these here.

Situations that worsen voices:

1.

2.

Can anybody else hear your voices?

The answer to this question is very important as it is a major determinant of the severity of the voices.

Most voice hearers have admitted that they have never really thought this question through. Most suspect that others can hear at least some of the voices or are unsure. As the voices can be nasty, or embarrassing, this causes anxiety when in public places, and for many voice hearers anxiety (worry, stress) makes the voices worse. We suggest that the best way to check this out is to speak to somebody you know and trust to check out whether that person can hear your voices. Good people to share this with might be a family member, your primary care physician, a close friend who knows about the problem, or a community psychiatric nurse or psychiatrist. It does mean taking that person into your confidence, but it is important to find out because if you don't need to worry about other people listening then you can do more social activities and hide away less. Another really good way to find out is to set up an experiment. Once the voices have started up switch on a tape recorder and see if those voices are recorded on the tape. If, when you replay the tape, those voices are not there then we can stop worrying about other people hearing.

Ask someone you trust and who knows about your illness the following question. "I hear voices that sound very real; if I tell you when I hear them will you tell me what you can hear?"

What is the explanation?

Marius Romme did a survey of voice hearers and found that those who were coping well had discovered that others couldn't hear the voice and had worked out a good explanation. Some good copers concluded that the voices were childhood memories, a special gift or ability to hear spirits, flashbacks of distressing experiences, or spiritual messages of encouragement. Fiona concluded that her voices were probably related to a period of time before she lost her job when her husband was very nasty to her when he was drinking heavily. He said lots of things to her that he wouldn't have said when sober but they hurt her very deeply. Fiona was able to conclude the following:

1. Nobody else can hear my voices no matter how loud or nasty they are, so I will never run away from them.
2. My ex-husband was so nasty to me that my brain couldn't cope and I still hear his comments as voices (an echo of the past).

A voice diary is crucial: it can help us to begin to get some control by identifying quiet periods and some possible coping strategies. It can also help us to decide whether or not others can hear the voice and to decide on an explanation.

An example of a completed voice diary including coping strategies

Situation	Voice present?	What did voice say?	Loudness 1/10	How did I feel?	What did I do?
Cooking breakfast	No				
Getting dressed	Yes	She looks grubby	4/10	Ashamed	Said to myself "I look very fashionable." I put on some classical music.
At yoga class	Yes	Ha! Ha! She's with all her scum pals	8/10	Panic	Deep breathing "No one can hear."
Shopping	Yes	No one would fancy you	7/10	Sad	Looked people in the eye said to myself "I am a good person."

Voice diary and coping strategies template

Situation	Voice present?	What did voice say?	Loudness 1/10	How did I feel?	What did I do?
Write in your own activities over a day and try to do some different things.	Yes or no.	Write down some of the main things the voice was saying.	10/10 maximum 1/10 a whisper	Sad? Angry? Anxious? etc.	Use a coping strategy? Think better thoughts?

This second diary allows us to begin to see how the voice hearing causes certain feelings. People usually have the same sort of feelings when the voice comes on. Some people feel angry that their privacy is being invaded, or that they are being commented upon in a negative way, or that they are being given instructions. This is the kind of feeling that you get when you think you have not been treated fairly. As a strong emotion, anger usually makes voices louder and more distressing. Those people who get angry at the voices need to think about working on feeling more relaxed when the voices come on. As mentioned above some people feel ashamed. If they have tested it out and found that others can't hear, then they need to remind themselves of this.

How do I feel when the voice is speaking?

This is a very important question as people who are calm, relaxed, and who feel in control tend to have less troublesome voices.

Ashamed

This is the kind of feeling you get when you think others are thinking badly of you, e.g., do you remember that time in primary school when the teacher embarrassed you in front of the class? Feeling ashamed normally happens because in the back of your mind you still think that other people can hear your voices and might disapprove. Feeling ashamed makes you hide away from social meetings and makes the voices worse. You need to ask someone you trust "Can you hear this voice?" You then need to try to tape the voices. Then convinced in your own mind that only you can hear them go into public places and observe other people. Do they look as if they are hearing loud and nasty voices? If they did they would show some evidence, like all looking round to see where they were coming from. Finally talk yourself through it, "these voices are only meant for me!" "No one else can hear them . . . so they aren't judging me."

Anxiety

This is an unpleasant feeling of fright. There are worrying thoughts in the mind, butterflies in the tummy, shaking, sweating, finding it hard to breath, and palpitations of the heart. This unpleasant feeling is a common one for voice hearers and it usually makes the voices worse. Lots of things can help anxiety, e.g., deep breathing, use of relaxation exercises. Anxiety can be reduced by rational self-talk. An example is given below.

Voice: "Work is God's business . . . he will never work . . . the power is not with him." *Jim's thought about the voice:* "This is all too much . . . it is too strong for me . . . I'm a victim of a supernatural being."

Feeling strong anxiety, Jim hid away from normal life because of his fear. This made the voice worse. One way of talking back to such a voice is to tell the voice that you are boss! That no supernatural being would say such things and that it is only a trick of the mind. There is no danger and you will not obey. This means a revolution against the voices, and very often when you take on even an opponent who sounds strong you can win. Look at David and Goliath!

Anger

This is a strong emotion, which usually leads to trouble! Imagine yourself in a car park – you have waited for ten minutes for a parking space to become empty. A vicar drives in and sees you waiting but accelerates into the first space. How do you feel? You are probably furious. You are telling yourself that this is not fair . . . and him a man of the cloth as well. Often when we are angry the mind uses labels for people, e.g., "thoughtless bastard." Such negative labels only act to make you feel more angry. You then start to think that something must be done about this injustice. Once you have let all the air out of the vicar's tyres you notice that he has a pregnant woman in the car who is going into labour. Anger can be reduced by looking carefully at what is going on and talking yourself through it rationally. If you are angry at your voices you are probably telling yourself it isn't fair what the voice is saying and perhaps swearing at the voice. Tell yourself, the voice is part of me and I am going to work with it and not against it.

If we can identify our emotional reaction to the voice then we can start to work on any unhelpful emotions. This should help to reduce voice intensity and perhaps frequency.

What is my typical emotion when I hear the voice? Write it in here.

1.

2.

Safety behaviors

These seem to help for a short time, but very quickly act to keep voices going. Basically a safety behavior is what it says, it works to keep you safe from the voice(s). The most obvious one is staying in bed, but not going out of the house is another, and living in a cannabis or alcohol haze is another. These may help reduce how often we hear a voice, and may help us avoid some of the unpleasant emotions felt when we hear a voice. However, if we hide away then the voices don't have the chance to be tested in the real world and so tend to never change. Use the voice diary and put in some different and interesting things. Maybe things you used to be interested in but have given up. How about a bicycle ride . . . or reviving an old hobby like bird watching, or visiting some local historical sites, or going back to see the football team you used to support. What are your safety behaviors?

Write them in this space.

1.

2.

3.

Now give them up with the help of some of the coping strategies from the voice diary. What are you going to do to get back to normal?

1.

2.

3.

It can feel very difficult to give up these behaviors, because they help make us feel safe, and may reduce the frequency of hearing voices. However, people usually find that if they give up the behaviors, and go out more, or manage differently when out (i.e., not having smoked lots of cannabis), then actually the voice is no worse than normal, and sometimes can be even less noticeable.

Better coping strategies

As we give up the safety behaviors we will need even stronger coping strategies to help us cope. We need to know that there is something we can do to take the edge off the voices. Obviously, medication usually helps at least a bit in this area. Everyone needs to find a strategy that works for them because everybody is different. We need to try things out until we find what works for us. Why not work down the following list, giving each one a trial of a day to see if it is working?

1. Hum a tune or whistle . . . let's make it a tune to show our determination, how about *The Great Escape, Colonel Bogey, The Dambusters March,* or if you prefer *New York, New York* or *American Idiot.* Does it work? If it seems to be helping a bit then extend the trial period up to a full week.

2. Listen to music or an audio-book on a CD or cassette player and headphones. Usually the more interesting and relevant the recorded material, the more help it is. As before, if it seems to be helping a bit, then use it for a full week before giving up on it.

3. Take this book with you, and read this chapter when the voices come on.

4. Think of a very positive experience you have had, e.g., winning a prize at the school sports day or being given a compliment. Hold the image in your mind for a while, and let your mind dwell on it. How do the voices react?

5. Tell yourself that the voice has a personal meaning for you and that it is a positive force in your life even if it sounds negative.

6. Use a positive spiritual approach like a mantra or a prayer.

7. Talk back to the voices if the content of the voices is not true of you. If a voice is saying something that you know not to be true, it is important that you treat it as if it were a factual mistake, like if your name was spelt wrongly on an envelope. Just because a voice says something does not mean it is true!

8. Use your mobile phone but don't switch it on. Speak into the phone to tell the voice you can speak to it later and that you are in charge. If the voice says something negative then gently put it right by telling the voice the fact of the matter.

Getting some self-esteem

Voices very often feed off low self-esteem. If you believe that you are a bad person, or unlovable, or a failure, or a reject, then the voices will probably repeat this at length. So who are you and what is your worth? We should probably all ask ourselves these questions, because very often we have decided in childhood that we are "a loser" or "useless" when in actual fact we are OK.

Who are you? I am Douglas . . . childhood was good but dad did too much work and didn't like any kind of illness. I learned that you should work every hour God sends and if you get sick then you should be ashamed. I was well looked after and believed that I was basically OK.

What are you worth? As long as I am working all the time and don't get sick I have value as a person.

What is the fact of it? I am a decent person whether or not I am working or sick.

How can I come to believe this? By writing a letter, thinking it through, talking to others about it.

Answer the questions below.

Who am I?

What am I worth?

(If we can give ourselves some self-esteem then the voices may well back off a bit.)

What should I believe about myself?

1.

2.

3.

What can I do to build these views? It may be important to build up your sense of self-esteem by doing some of the activities you have avoided, as described above (like going to the football match, seeing a friend). If you can build on your strengths, and do more rewarding activities, you may hear the voices less as you are busy. You will most likely feel better about yourself and this will make any negative voice content less believable, because you will know that you are a good person with qualities and strengths. The voices may say something bad, but it does not mean they are true.

Cultural and religious aspects of voice hearing

Example 4

Ronnie was 24 years of age when he emigrated from Nigeria with his mother to work in the UK. Initially, things did not go as smoothly for him as planned, as he was experiencing difficulties in getting a job and overall in adjusting to life in a different country. He had left all his friends behind and missed them. He started hearing the voice of his grandfather telling him "You are useless. You cannot do anything right." The voice also started telling him "People do not like you here. You will never get a job." As the voice became more frequent and criticized everything he did, he started feeling down about these comments and told his mother, who explained to him that his experience was normal and "sometimes ancestors guide us in life." With time, he started believing what the voice was saying to him and slowly started withdrawing into himself. He stopped eating, going out, and thought he was worthless, and that people were against him.

In some cultures, it can be acceptable and a positive experience to communicate with ancestors. However, when these experiences make it harder to function and carry on with daily tasks, then it is worth looking at what is causing the distress. It is also worth considering that managing the voices may reduce the distress and improve life. In Ronnie's case, stress had probably triggered the voice that was distressing him. As it can be acceptable in some cultures for ancestors to guide people, his mother did not encourage him to get help. The aim of getting help is not to challenge cultural beliefs, but to work with the distress.

Summary

1. Voice experiences are common and most people will have such an experience in their lives. Hearing voices is not a sign that someone is ill or mad, rather it is a normal experience.
2. Some people, such as spiritualists or mediums, perceive their voices in a positive way. They consider them to be a gift. Other people will value their voice experiences as they can provide companionship and comfort.
3. Hence, it is not the presence of a voice in itself that is the problem, it is the attitude we take towards it, and how it makes us feel and react or behave.
4. Keeping a diary will help identify any patterns to the voice experiences: you can then increase activities that are associated with hearing the voices less, and try and reduce periods when you do hear voices (e.g., being alone, watching a dull film on TV). This will help give you some control.
5. If a voice says something that you do not agree with, or is not true, you do not have to believe it. If it is not true of you, does it really matter what it says?

6. Try and test out whether others can hear your voice too.
7. Try and increase the positive or rewarding activities that you do; this will help you feel better.
8. Try and reduce or stop the safety behaviors; they may not actually be needed.
9. Try new coping strategies, such as the ones described here or others that you have found useful.
10. Build your self-esteem, build on your strengths.

5

Overcoming negative symptoms

Ron Siddle

Overview

This chapter aims to offer the reader an understanding of negative symptoms, such as low motivation and blunting of emotions. Techniques are described to help gradually lift these distressing symptoms.

Chapter contents

- What are negative symptoms?
- Describing negative symptoms
- Do you have negative symptoms?
- Distinguishing between negative symptoms and other difficulties
- Causes of negative symptoms
- Primary negative symptoms
- Secondary negative symptoms
- The consequences of having negative symptoms
- What about my family?
- Education
- Grading your tasks
- Activity scheduling
- Points to note
- Cultural and religious aspects
- Summary

What are negative symptoms?

Psychiatrists often describe schizophrenia as including both positive and negative symptoms. Positive symptoms are symptoms, such as voices and paranoia, that people with schizophrenia have, and which most people without schizophrenia do not have. Negative symptoms, on the other hand, involve symptoms in which the person has a deficit in some aspect of their normal functioning: these can be found in people without schizophrenia.

It may be that you do not have schizophrenia, but even if that is the case, it won't do any harm to give you some information about this group of symptoms that can also be found in people without schizophrenia.

Describing negative symptoms

Negative symptoms include the following.

Alogia relates to impoverished thinking and can be characterized by *poverty of speech (reduced speech)*. Other symptoms include *thought blocking*, an increase in the time taken to respond when asked questions. The person themselves may not notice this symptom, but family members or friends might.

Anergia is a lack of energy or drive. People with anergia may be unable to motivate themselves, possibly resulting in poor hygiene, occupational difficulties, and drastically reduced levels of social functioning. People can suffer deterioration in performance and may spend hours without any spontaneous activity. This can have disastrous consequences for people in employment or those taking further education.

Anhedonia is a symptom where people have difficulty in experiencing pleasure or taking enjoyment from recreational pursuits, friendships, or sexual relationships. Some people with these symptoms find it difficult to express intimacy with others and have difficulty developing and maintaining relationships with friends or colleagues.

Emotional blunting is where the person has difficulty experiencing and demonstrating emotion, and this can also cause difficulty in maintaining relationships. With this symptom, people can show unchanging facial expressions and may fail to make appropriate eye contact. Both of these have an effect upon building and maintaining relationships.

In many cases, attention and concentration may also be impaired and the person may be unable to think in abstract terms, being able only to display a fixed or concrete thinking style. This is why psychiatrists often ask people about proverbs, because people who think concretely often struggle to understand the secondary meaning implicit in the proverb.

Do you have negative symptoms?

Since trying to detect the absence of a characteristic is often harder than detecting the presence of a characteristic this may be difficult.

Nonetheless, it may be worthwhile trying to see if you have any of the symptoms above. You might also ask someone whose judgment you trust, to give their view.

Symptom	Your assessment	Trusted other
Alogia		
Anergia		
Anhedonia		
Emotional blunting		
Concrete thinking		

Negative symptoms are important for a number of reasons. Why do you think negative symptoms might be important to you?

1.

2.

3.

You may have your own reasons why negative symptoms are important. You might not know that negative symptoms are also important because:

1. Research has shown that they can have an effect upon a person's outcome from treatment (in other words how well they respond to treatment).
2. Negative symptoms can also have an unhelpful effect upon therapeutic interventions used in treating positive symptoms of schizophrenia.
3. Researchers who have explored family relationships inform us that it is often negative symptoms that cause annoyance and irritation in family members. Though this is in itself something we may wish to avoid, the research shows that excessive criticism from family members can also influence the person's risk of having a relapse.

Distinguishing between negative symptoms and other difficulties: causes of confusion

Depression is a common mental health difficulty and many people experience the illness of depression, while almost all of us have been unhappy at some time in our lives. It is said that up to half of people who have schizophrenia also experience symptoms of depression. Although the features of depression and negative symptoms can overlap, there is a difference between depression and negative symptoms, and if you are troubled with the symptoms mentioned above, it may be helpful to establish that your symptoms are truly negative symptoms, and not depression. The hallmark of depression is of course a very deep sadness often accompanied by insomnia, lack of appetite, and loss of libido. Another major source of confusion with negative symptoms is neuroleptic-induced deficit syndrome, which sometimes occurs as a side effect of some antipsychotic medication. The features of neuroleptic-induced deficit syndrome are sometimes called pseudo-parkinsonism and can be misinterpreted as either depressive symptoms, negative symptoms of schizophrenia, or both. This sounds complicated and it can be difficult to work it out, so it is often best to ask your psychiatrist or primary care physician.

Causes of negative symptoms

It would be fair to say that we are not absolutely certain of the cause or causes of negative symptoms. Some people believe that they are a result of biological changes in the brain, while others believe that negative symptoms are a response to stressful situations. Psychiatrists generally believe that there are two kinds of negative symptoms. Primary negative symptoms are thought to be the product of a biological illness process, while secondary negative symptoms can be thought of as a natural result of positive symptoms such as hallucinations.

Primary negative symptoms: a biological view

Biologists describe negative symptoms resulting from a loss of brain cells and from structural changes in the brain, which are associated with an illness process.

Secondary negative symptoms: a psychological view

On the other hand, if a man was lying in bed all day because he heard a voice telling him he was to be killed if he went out of the house, this might be considered to be a secondary negative symptom. According to this view, negative symptoms are a response to difficult psychological and social situations – and can be considered to be a coping strategy against stress. The person's withdrawal from social situations and their reduced activity is a protective feature against further difficulties. The secondary negative symptoms are thought to be far more temporary and more easily treatable than primary negative symptoms, although it may be difficult to distinguish between these two types.

> If you have negative symptoms, can you think of any reasons why you might have developed them?

The consequences of having negative symptoms

Negative symptoms can have a profound effect on your quality of life. Because your communication may be affected if you have negative symptoms, relationships with family members and friends can suffer. Because of negative symptoms you may give up hobbies and pastimes, and you may lose your job, which may also reduce the amount of intellectual stimulation and human contact, and even affect your financial income.

As if these risks were not bad enough, relatives or friends may complain about your lack of responsiveness, or they can criticize you for being lazy, which you might be aware of and be concerned about.

Symptoms such as poverty of speech and reduced content of speech may distance you from normal and enjoyable social interactions, while lack of energy may deny you the opportunity to engage in pleasurable activities or feel a sense of reward from tackling successful projects. Reduction in concentration can have an additional and unhelpful effect upon the chances of you obtaining feelings of satisfaction from a successful job completed, pleasure, or of successful social interaction. In addition to all of these difficulties, the stigma associated with schizophrenia, and financial constraints, could have an effect upon an individual's willingness and ability to join in social events.

What about my family?

Family studies have shown that negative symptoms are a source of distress for family and carers, with many relatives believing that the behavior described earlier is because of laziness. Family members can also experience feelings of "burden" because of the reduction in domestic and self-care activity resulting from the negative symptoms. This can result in a belief that the family are "doing more than their fair share", and in family members reducing their own social activities and their own personal relationships, outside the home. This can be an additional source of stress, dissatisfaction, and disagreement within the whole family unit (see Chapter 9).

What have been the consequences for you of negative symptoms?

If you have not had difficulties from negative symptoms try to consider others with more serious difficulties who may have been troubled by severe negative symptoms. What problems might they have?

Education

Negative symptoms can be as widely misunderstood as hallucinations and delusions. You and, where appropriate, your family members can think of the lack of activity, emotional blunting, and restricted communication as unhelpful and wilful personal characteristics rather than illness-related symptoms. Sufferers are at times described as "lazy", "not bothered," or "negligent of their responsibilities." These descriptions can contribute to negative attitudes and critical behavior towards the sufferer, which can reinforce a poor self-image in the person himself or herself (see Chapter 8).

Information about the symptoms and how they relate to the course of the illness is needed, as well as an explanation of how these behaviors relate to the positive symptoms of schizophrenia. People also need to understand the long time scale that is likely to be needed to make an impact on these problems. Work in this area needs to be seen in terms of months and years rather than weeks and months – but people need to be aware that definite progress can be made. Many psychiatric services have staff trained in psychosocial interventions (PSI) who might be able to help your family to get a better idea about these and other symptoms, as it can be hard for you to explain such symptoms particularly when you are being criticized.

Some of the CBT approaches used in the treatment of depression might also be used in the treatment of some of your negative symptoms. By increasing your activity levels, it can be possible to increase feelings of reward (achievement), pleasure, or both. Assuming that you want to work with these areas, a number of specific CBT techniques might be helpful.

Grading your tasks

Sometimes the activities and tasks ahead can appear overwhelming and feelings of demoralization can quickly take over. Grading tasks involves the breaking down of tasks or skills into their component parts. The component parts could be time segments as in an example such as digging a garden, where you might carry out ten minutes of digging then take a well-earned break. Alternatively, it could be split into logical components, such as digging a row and then having a break.

For this technique to be of value, the task that you wish to complete, for example, tidy the lounge, would be broken down into components that were readily achievable and in which each chunk was possible within your concentration span allowing for breaks and rewards between the component parts.

Grading a task

Assume that you have decided to paint your room. Write down the stages of this task.
Stages that we considered were:
- Roughly guesstimate the amount of paint needed and write a list
- Go and buy the paint
- Empty the room
- Sand the woodwork (may be further broken down if too large)
- Undercoat wood
- Paint ceiling
- Paint wall 1
- Paint wall 2
- Paint wall 3
- Paint wall 4
- Paint woodwork
- Move furniture back

How did you do? As you might imagine, a big job like this will take a long time and it's important not to give up or to try to do too much at one go, otherwise you might sicken yourself. Now let's try another graded task assignment.

Graded task assignment

Write down a task that you would like to do, but have been putting off for so long because it's too big.

Now break down this task into manageable chunks.

Why not discuss this with a family member or health care professional, to see that you have not bitten off more than you can chew?

Activity scheduling

People who keep busy have more opportunities for satisfying and pleasurable activities than those who do not. It is recognized that people with negative symptoms have more difficulties with energy levels, but it is still worthwhile looking at this technique used by health workers in depression, as it increases the opportunities for satisfaction and pleasure, which must be worth trying for. There are essentially three types of activity that seem to characterize most of our day-to-day activities.

These are as follows.

- *Pleasure activities* are those things that we simply enjoy doing – we enjoy these activities for their own merits. There need not be any skill involved in these activities. Examples could include: eating chocolates, watching TV, having a beer, having a bath, and so forth.
- *Reward activities* are those that are not necessarily pleasurable, but the person achieves a sense of satisfaction when the activity is done. There might be a degree of skill or a need to get yourself motivated to do these. Reward activities might include: having a bet on the horses, gardening, DIY, playing the guitar, etc.
- *Chores* can be pleasurable, involve a sense of reward, or can be simply tasks that a person feels obliged to do. For some people they might give no sense

of pleasure or reward, while for others they might be very pleasurable and rewarding. Examples might include: taking the kids to school, paying the bills, or washing up dishes.

Write down the activities that you think are pleasurable.

Did they all involve cost? Now reexamine your list and add to it things that give pleasure that don't cost anything.

Some ideas here might include:
- watching your favorite films on a (borrowed) DVD or video
- taking your nephews for a walk in the park
- hot soak in the bath with relaxing music
- picnic in your favorite spot
- going for a bike ride.

As you can see it's not all expensive. Most of us have different proportions of pleasurable, rewarding, and chore type activities, though depressed people are known to have a tendency to gradually eliminate both reward and pleasure activities. You can imagine what life would be like if it had only chores and lots of opportunities to sit and think about how awful life is. In many people, a reasonable aim might be to increase reward and pleasure activities.

What proportion of your time do you think is spent on the following activities?
- Reward
- Pleasure
- Chores
- Doing none of these e.g., sitting and thinking

In order to gain an accurate idea about your activity pattern it can be useful to gather data for a few days or ideally longer. To do this, look at the table below, which allows the day to be split into hour-long periods. You should record the main activity during that hour, and how you would rate it in terms of reward and pleasure. For example let's assume you got up at 9 am, and between 9 am and 10 am you showered and ate breakfast. You could write either activity, both activities, or the most important one. Then the activities would be rated out of ten, with 0/10 being not rewarding or not pleasurable, while 10/10 would be very rewarding or very pleasurable. Bear in mind that some activities may score highly on both reward and pleasure, some will score low on both, and some will be high on one while low on the other. In the example mentioned earlier, the rating recorded by this person was:

Time	Activity	Rating Reward and pleasure
8–9 am	Showering Breakfast	R = 4/10 P = 0/10 R = 1/10 P = 8/10

Activity plan template

Time	Activity	Rating Reward and pleasure

So, what is the point of this?

Once you have started recording your activities, you must, of course, review them and see if your activity levels might be adding to your difficulties and work out if they could be altered. Keeping fairly accurate records (as opposed to remembering the most memorable events in the past week) allows us to see how we fill our days and see what activities we do that give us a bit of a buzz. Then, we can alter our activity plans to do more of these. This is, of course, the whole point of the recording, to highlight to you what you are doing and which activities you ought to increase and which you ought to reduce. As an example, if you noticed that you got a sense of reward from tidying up the garden, it might be worth trying to do that a bit more often, or at times when you were feeling more miserable than others. After all, most of us would get benefit from doing more rewarding things. As a bonus, the more time you can fill with activities leaves less time to sit and worry or dwell upon things, which most people rate as adding to their troubles.

So, the order we suggest for doing this is to keep records for a couple of days to see how things are right now. Then, review the patterns and see which are helpful activities and which are not helping. For almost all of us sitting and thinking too much is unhelpful, but there may be other activities that are very helpful, e.g., when you go to visit your brother. Once you are aware of your own helpful and unhelpful activities, you need to plan to increase the helpful activities and minimize the unhelpful activities. You may not be able to avoid the unhelpful ones completely, but perhaps you can schedule them for when you are feeling better, e.g., if you are a morning person do them then. You might also want to ask yourself if you really do need to do the activity. Some of the time we believe that we really must do things, when there is no law that says we have to.

Points to note

Set yourself short-term achievable goals, which allow you to develop a sense of achievement. If you have negative symptoms, then you are likely to have a serious illness and it may not be possible to immediately get up and do all that you want to do. Think of increasing your activity levels as a marathon rather than a sprint.

Care is clearly needed to ensure that you are not overloaded, and no matter how keen you are to get back to college or work, try to ensure that a number of purely pleasurable activities are included for each day or activity period. You must not forget to plan pleasurable activities when you are planning your other activities, as some people try too hard and end up overloading themselves.

The plan breaks the day into smaller, sometimes hourly, segments. Tasks, activities, and rest periods are built into the plan in a way that enables you to balance your day, which is more likely to result in pleasure or a sense of reward and accomplishment or both.

Where negative symptoms are more severe, your aims and objectives should be modest. Some people may derive more benefit from having a predictable pattern to their day, while others would prefer more variety in their activities from one day to the next. Your task is to decide how best to achieve this, since for some people a weekly activity plan might be too daunting, while for others the prospect of a plan is very reassuring. Remember that even though we might hope that you will develop a plan, we do hope and expect that the plan can and should be altered if an opportunity arises to do something more rewarding or more pleasurable than that which was scheduled.

This is an area where relatives or friends could be particularly helpful, by helping you to detect patterns in the activity records, and by encouraging limited but achievable goals, helping you to identify and overcome obstacles so that a sense of accomplishment is achieved. Relatives could be involved in monitoring progress, offering an appropriate level of stimulation or prompting, and most importantly in the giving of praise or rewards for efforts made.

There is an issue with this that we are sure you will have realized by now. All this takes effort and may not work for you, but we hope that you are now aware of how these techniques can possibly help and are willing to give it a try. You should perhaps set yourself a goal and make sure it's reasonable, then try monitoring your activities for a while and finally try to change your activities for a while. If that does not help, you will have wasted a few sheets of paper and some effort, but surely the potential benefits would make this a worthwhile risk.

Jot down all of the potential benefits of these techniques if they are successful.

Now jot down all of the costs of trying these techniques.

Is it worth a try?

Cultural and religious aspects

Case study

Ram is a 28-year-old Indian man who lives with his parents. Culturally it is normal for Ram to live with his parents even though some may consider that he is old enough to be independent. His mother continues to cook meals for him and do his washing, and he in turn has always looked after his parents when they have been unwell. Ram developed schizophrenia at the age of 22. With medication and help from the mental health services his positive symptoms have been well controlled. However, his mother has noticed recently that even though she does his washing, he is reluctant to even give her his laundry. She has also complained that he is not as compassionate with his parents anymore when they are unwell. His care coordinator from the mental health services recognized the problem and has been working on Ram's negative symptoms. He has also explained the problem to Ram's parents.

This example highlights that negative symptoms can occur across cultures. Some may have considered Ram to be lazy, as his mother did his laundry and cooking. This was culturally normal for Ram. It was the change in his level of activity, interest, and emotional response that signified his negative symptoms.

Summary

1. Negative symptoms are likely to have a number of effects upon a person's domestic and social life.
2. Techniques and strategies are suggested to minimize and reduce the consequences of these symptoms.
3. By using these approaches, it may be possible to help you to overcome your difficulties more effectively.

FURTHER READING

Andreason, N. C. (1989). The scale for the assessment of negative symptoms (SANS): conceptual and theoretical foundations. *British Journal of Psychiatry*, **155,** 49–52.

Barnes, T. R. E. (1994). Issues in the clinical assessment of negative symptoms. *Current Opinion in Psychiatry*, **7**, 35–8.

Barnes, T. R. E. & Liddle, P. F. (1990). Evidence for the validity of negative symptoms. In N. C. Andreasen, ed., *Schizophrenia: Positive and Negative Symptoms and Syndromes*, Vol. 24. Basel: Karger, pp. 43–72.

Barnes, T. R. E., Curzon, D. A., Liddle, P. F. & Patel, M. (1989). The nature and prevalence of depression in chronic schizophrenic in-patients. *British Journal of Psychiatry*, **154**, 486–91.

Barrowclough, C. & Tarrier, N. (1992). *Families of Schizophrenic Patients: Cognitive Behavioural Interventions.* London: Chapman and Hall.

Birchwood, M., Smith, J., Cochrane, R., Wetton, S. & Copestake, S. (1990). The Social Functioning Scale: the development and validation of a scale of social adjustment for use in family intervention programmes with schizophrenic patients. *British Journal of Psychiatry*, **157**, 853–9.

Carpenter, W. T. Jr., Heinrichs, D. W. & Wagman, A. M. (1988). Deficit and non-deficit forms of schizophrenia. *American Journal of Psychiatry*, **145**, 578–83.

Crow, T. J. (1980). Molecular pathology of schizophrenia: more than one dimension of pathology. *British Medical Journal*, **143**, 66–8.

Fenton, W. S. & McGlashan, T. H., (1994). Antecedents, symptom progression, and long-term outcome of the deficit syndrome in schizophrenia. *American Journal of Psychiatry*, **151**(3), 351–6.

Hamilton, M. (1978). *Fish's Outline of Psychiatry*, 3rd edn. Bristol: John Wright.

Hogg, L. (1996). Psychological treatments for negative symptoms. In G. Haddock & P. Slade, eds., *Cognitive Behavioural Interventions with Psychosis.* London: Routledge.

Krawiecka, M., Goldberg, D. & Vaughan, M. (1977). A standardised psychiatric assessment rating for chronic psychotic patients. *Acta Psychiatrica Scandinavica*, **55**, 299–308.

Leff, J. (1990). Depressive symptoms in the course of schizophrenia. In L. E. DeLisi, ed., *Depression in Schizophrenia.* Washington: American Psychiatric Press, pp. 1–23.

Liddle, P. (1987). The symptoms of chronic schizophrenia: a re-examination of the positive–negative dichotomy. *British Journal of Psychiatry*, **151**, 145–51.

McKenna, P. J., Lund, C. E. & Mortimer, A. M. (1989). Negative symptoms: relationship to other schizophrenic symptom classes. *British Journal of Psychiatry*, **155** (suppl 7), 104–7.

Premack, D. (1975). Reinforcement theory. In A. E. Kazdin, ed., *Behavior Modification in Applied Settings.* Homewood, IL: The Dorsey Press.

Thara, R. & Eaton, W. W. (1996). Outcome of schizophrenia: the Madras longitudinal study. *Australian and New Zealand Journal of Psychiatry*, **30**, 516–22.

6

Tablets and injections

Richard Gray

Overview

This chapter aims to offer the reader an understanding of the role of antipsychotic medicines in facilitating recovery and preventing relapse. The importance of clear communication between patient and doctor is stressed in order that compliance might be optimized.

- Cultural and religious aspects
- Summary

This book has focused on a range of self-help techniques to help you manage your psychosis. For many people medication is an important part of managing psychosis. Many people think that self-help and talking therapies work best when people are also taking some medication to help with their psychosis. This chapter is all about the tablets and injections that are available for psychosis. We believe that having control over your medication is just as important as having control over *your* psychosis. So the aim of this chapter is to help you:
- talk to your health professional
- choose the medication that is best for you
- manage your medication to get the most out of it.

Reflection about medication

Before doing any detailed work about your medication it is often helpful to begin with some quiet reflection. Take ten minutes to think about and write down your experiences of antipsychotic medication. Write down the medications or treatments that have been helpful as well as those that have not been so helpful. Then think about how you would like things to be different with your medication. For example, would you have liked more information about the different types of medication, or would you like to have tried alternatives to medication?

Exercise 1

Take ten minutes to think about and write down your experiences of medication. Try not to write a list but write thoughts and ideas around the cloud as they occur to you.

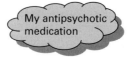

Exercise 2

Take ten minutes to think about and write down how you would like things to be different with your antipsychotic medication. Again try not to write a list but write thoughts and ideas around the cloud as they occur to you.

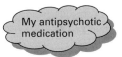

Talking to psychiatrists, family doctors, and health professionals

Talking to health professionals can be very difficult, as meetings often have strict time limits and it can be hard to assert yourself and express your concerns. The key to getting what you want out of any meeting with a professional is to be prepared. Think in advance about what your aim for the meeting is and try and stick to it. We have listed some "power questions" that you might find useful when talking to health professionals.

"Power questions" are essential and focused questions to ask during a meeting with a health professional. Having a set of questions can prepare you for the meeting so that you get the most out of your time. It can also help you feel more involved in the decisions about your care and treatment.

Listed below are a number of power questions that might help focus the discussions. These are just suggestions (although you may want to photocopy this page and take it to the meeting with you); you may choose to make up your own. Before the meeting write down the questions you want answered and work through them one by one. You could say to the health professional: "I have some questions about my medication that are important to me. I need to go through them with you now."

Examples of power questions are as follows:

Starting an antipsychotic

1. What choice of medication is available to me?

2. How do they work?

3. How effective are they?

4. What symptoms will it help?

Getting the full picture

1. What side effects are associated with this medication?

2. What is the best way to manage them?

3. How long will I have to take the medication?

4. What will happen if/when I stop it?

Other considerations

1. Do I need any special blood tests/health checks while I am taking it?

2. How often will the medication be reviewed?

3. What choice of other treatments is available to me?

4. If I choose not to take medication what other choices are available to me?

Excercise 3

Take ten minutes to think about what you know and what you want to know about the antipsychotic medication you are taking or thinking of taking.

1. What do you currently know about psychosis?

2. What do you currently know about your antipsychotic medication choices?

3. What additional information do you want about psychosis?

4. What additional information do you want about antipsychotic medication?

What do I need to know?

Power questions are very useful and will help you get more out of meetings with mental health professionals. There may well be additional information that you want about psychosis and antipsychotic medication. Exercise 3 is about identifying what you know and what you want to know about your medication. The information in this chapter may help *you* answer some of the questions but you may also want to discuss the questions with a mental health professional.

What is psychosis?

Let us look at the different experiences that people with psychosis have to deal with. This is important because different medicines may help with different experiences that doctors call symptoms. What you think your main symptom is will affect which medicine you should think about taking.

Altered experiences

Psychosis is a term used by doctors to describe a wide range of altered experiences. For example, some people may hear voices in their head when there is no one around; others may have distressing beliefs that cause them extreme concern and upset (for example, that they are being followed by the police or that they caused a plane crash). Doctors call these experiences positive symptoms. They are called positive symptoms because they are experiences added to the person not because they are good. Psychotic experiences can seem very real and be very distressing and upsetting. There are some other experiences that people with psychosis can have. These include:

- difficulty getting on with day-to-day things (negative symptoms – where something has been taken away from the person)
- thinking (cognitive symptoms)
- mood symptoms (depression and mania).

Positive symptoms of psychosis

The main "positive" symptoms of psychosis are:

- hallucinations (hearing voices, seeing visions, having a bad taste in your mouth, smelling bad things, or having the feeling that you are being touched)
- delusions (a strongly held belief in something that is not shared by people in your culture)
- thought disorder (problems in communicating, for example, during conversations, jumping from topic to topic).

Difficulty getting on with day-to-day things (negative symptoms)

People who have psychotic symptoms sometimes find it hard to get on with day-to-day things like getting up in the morning, getting washed and dressed, and cooking and cleaning. People may also feel detached from the world and may not seem to enjoy things – watching TV, playing sport, going shopping – the way they used to. Doctors sometimes call these negative symptoms. It is not that people have become lazy. These symptoms can happen when people have psychosis.

Getting on with people

Relationships with family and friends can sometimes be affected in people with psychosis. People may feel that they don't or can't talk to people that are close to them.

Thinking (cognitive symptoms)

People with psychosis can also have difficulty with their thinking. Sometimes people have problems concentrating (for example watching a film all the way through) or sorting out practical problems (such as dealing with money or planning a meal). Doctors call these cognitive symptoms. Difficulty with thinking can get in the way of work and occupation, and can be a real problem for many people with psychosis.

Mood (mood symptoms)

Sometimes people with psychosis can have a low mood or even become depressed. Often this is because of the distressing nature of some of their experiences (such as hearing voices saying bad things about them). Sometimes people can also become elated or high. Doctors call this symptom "mania."

What do you think?

What do you think about this description of the symptoms of psychosis? Everyone will experience psychosis differently. The symptoms of psychosis can make people angry and frustrated, especially when other people – particularly those close to them – don't believe that these experiences are real. What is the most problematic symptom for you?

Target symptom

Before we start talking about antipsychotic medicine let's begin by working out what you think is the main symptom or symptoms you experience that you want help with. Why don't you complete Exercise 4 (you could also do this exercise with help from a member of your family or your mental health professional). This exercise should help you work out what your main target symptom(s) are. We can then consider which antipsychotic medicine (if any) is going to be best for you.

Excercise 4

Identifying a target symptom

Step 1. Tick one circle for each item that best describes your symptoms over the last month.

	Not at all	Some of the time	Most of the time
1. Altered experiences (e.g., hearing voices, unusual beliefs)	○	○	○
2. Problems getting on with day-to-day things	○	○	○
3. Problems getting on with people	○	○	○
4. Thinking problems	○	○	○
5. Mood problems	○	○	○
6. Feeling angry	○	○	○

Step 2. Which of the symptoms that you are currently experiencing do you consider to be the main problem? Try and describe your experiences in a few words in the box below.

My main problem is . . .

Harvey: identifying target symptoms

Harvey had heard voices for over five years. Initially they were nice voices that said kind and comforting things to him. Over the years the voices have become more critical, and Harvey has found them increasingly difficult to deal with. Over the past couple of years he has become increasingly withdrawn and found it harder to get up in the morning. He spends most of the day watching TV. He lives with his mum who looks after him. When Harvey did the identifying target symptoms exercise he said that he had altered experiences most of the time but he could "deal with the voice." However, he said that his main problem was getting on with day-to-day things because he was fed up with his mum "getting on his case."

What is antipsychotic medication?

Antipsychotic medication is, as the name suggests, medication that works against (anti) psychosis. There are lots of different types of antipsychotic medication. The older medicines are called typical (or sometimes conventional or first generation) antipsychotics and the newer ones atypical (or second generation) antipsychotics. Tables 6.1 and 6.2 list some of the commonly prescribed typical and atypical antipsychotics that are available (the information in these tables is adapted from the 2005–6 *Maudsley Prescribing Guidelines*). To give you an idea about how much of a medication you should be taking we have listed the minimum and maximum amount of medication that should be prescribed for people (aged 18–65) experiencing psychosis for the first time and for those who have had more than one period of psychosis. Different people need different doses of medication; this is because everyone's body deals with medication differently. Children and older adults (people over the age of 65) need less medication than working-age adults.

You will notice that a different amount of each medication is recommended (for example 800 mg per day of sulpiride is recommended as the minimum effective dose compared to 5 mg per day of haloperidol). This is to do with how strong the medicine is. So, for example, 2 mg per day of risperidone is about as strong as 150 mg per day of quetiapine. It is important that you get the right amount of medication.

Table 6.1 Conventional antipsychotics

Name	Minimum effective dose (first time taking antipsychotic medication)	Minimum effective dose (more than one episode of psychosis)	Maximum dose
Chlorpromazine	200 mg daily	300 mg daily	1000 mg daily
Haloperidol	2 mg daily	5 mg daily	30 mg daily
Sulpiride	400 mg daily	800 mg daily	2400 mg daily
Trifluoperazine	10 mg daily	15 mg daily	50 mg daily

Table 6.2 Atypical antipsychotics

Name	Minimum effective dose (first time taking antipsychotic medication)	Minimum effective dose (more than one episode of psychosis)	Maximum dose
Amisulpiride	400 mg daily	800 mg daily	1200 mg daily
Aripiprazole	10 mg daily	10 mg daily	30 mg daily
Clozapine (only for people who have got no benefit from other antipsychotics)	–	300 mg daily	900 mg daily
Olanzapine	5 mg daily	10 mg daily	20 mg daily
Quetiapine	150 mg daily	300 mg daily	800 mg daily
Risperidone	2 mg daily	4 mg daily	16 mg daily

Pills and injections

Most people take their antipsychotic medication as a pill or tablet. Different antipsychotic medications come in different formulations (ways of taking the drug):
- tablets or pills (the most common way of taking medication)
- tablets that dissolve in the mouth
- liquids or syrups
- injections given into muscle (normally your bottom)
- long-acting injections given into muscle (normally your bottom).

Some people take antipsychotic medication as a long-acting injection. Long-acting injections are often called "Depots." Depots are injected into the

Table 6.3 Depot and long-acting antipsychotics

Name	Minimum and maximum doses	How often is the injection given
Flupenthixol decanoate (Depixol)	12.5–400 mg	Every 2–4 weeks
Fluphenazine decanoate (Modecate)	6.25–50 mg	Every 2–5 weeks
Zuclopenthixol decanoate (Clopixol)	100–600 mg	Every 4 weeks
Risperidone long-acting injection (Risperdal Consta)	25, 37.5, or 50 mg	Every 2 weeks

large muscle in the bottom or thigh; when administered by a skilled mental health nurse the injection is generally not painful. Risperidone is the only atypical antipsychotic that is available as a long-acting injection. Depot medication can seem invasive and may not suit everyone. However, for some people it is a convenient way of taking antipsychotic medication. Table 6.3 shows the most often used long-acting injections.

A short-acting injection – doctors and nurses only give antipsychotic medication like this when someone is very distressed, violent, or aggressive to help them calm down. The drug is injected into the person's bottom. Most of the time medication is given like this as a one-off.

Liquids and dissolving tablets – some people find it hard to swallow tablets (or they don't like the taste). Some antipsychotic drugs can be given as a liquid or as a tablet that dissolves in your mouth – and some people prefer this.

Sally: choosing a long-acting injection

Sally became very paranoid after smoking cannabis while at college. Risperidone helped a lot with her paranoia and she was able to go back to college. However, Sally said "I forget to take medication three or four times a week, not on purpose I just forget." Because she missed medication she started to become more paranoid. She talked to her psychiatrist who started her on a long-acting injection of risperidone (Risperdal Consta). This worked well for Sally and kept her paranoia under control.

How does antipsychotic medication work?

Doctors think that symptoms of psychosis are caused by a chemical imbalance in people's brains. The brain chemical that is not balanced in people with psychosis is a chemical called dopamine. Too much dopamine in people's brains causes an increase in electrical activity in the emotional center of

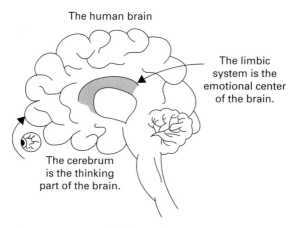

Figure 6.1 Diagram of the brain showing the limbic system, the main site of medication action

the brain; the emotional center of the brain is called the limbic region (see Figure 6.1). Increased electrical activity in this part of the brain seems to cause psychotic altered experiences, like hearing voices or feeling paranoid. A lack of dopamine in the part of the brain we use for thinking and processing information, the cerebrum, seems to cause difficulty in getting on with day-to-day things and problems in thinking (see Figure 6.1).

Can I stop antipsychotic medication once I feel better?

Often when we are ill we need to take a "course of treatment." For example, if you have a sore throat you may need a two-week course of antibiotics to get rid of the infection. Some illnesses are long term. Asthma is a long-term illness. Most people who have asthma need to take medication to get rid of their symptoms (e.g., breathing difficulties or coughing) and then need to keep taking medication to stop those symptoms from coming back. Psychosis is like asthma. You need to take medication to reduce or get rid of symptoms, and keep taking it to protect you from symptoms coming back.

Aimee: "I can stop medication when I feel better"

Aimee was 34 and had recently started believing that she was being controlled by alien beings that lived in the TV and radio. She was prescribed aripiprazole by her psychiatrist that she took for six weeks. She said that the belief about being controlled had "gone away" and she said she was "better." Aimee thought that because she was better she could stop taking her medication. After a couple of months the belief that she was being controlled by aliens started to return. The nurse that she was working with explained the importance of taking medication for at least two years to stop the experiences coming back. She started aripiprazole again and has been taking it fairly regularly for six months. The beliefs have not come back.

Effects against psychotic altered experiences (or positive symptoms)

Antipsychotic medication works against altered experiences by slowing electrical activity in the limbic region of the brain. About eight out of ten people who have psychotic altered experiences say that medication helps. Often these experiences don't go away completely, but they may become less frequent, intense, or distressing. Because of improvements in psychotic experiences people may feel less agitated and angry; some also find that they get on better with family and friends. These are the indirect positive effects of antipsychotic medication.

Emily: "the indirect benefits of antipsychotic medication"

Emily was 22 years old and had been hearing very distressing voices telling her she was "an evil person" and should "kill herself." She had had these experiences for about six months before she went to see her family doctor. Emily was convinced that the voice she heard was her dead mother talking from "beyond the grave." Emily's dad was very distressed by Emily's experiences and they argued a lot about her experiences. Emily's family doctor prescribed her an antipsychotic medication called sulpiride. After two weeks of taking sulpiride Emily said that the voice she heard had "faded into the background" and didn't bother her as much. Emily's relationship with her dad improved dramatically and for both Emily and her dad this was the most important positive effect of antipsychotic medication.

Effects against negative symptoms and thinking problems

Conventional antipsychotic medication is really only effective against altered experiences or positive symptoms of psychosis. The new antipsychotic drugs (atypical) seem to also be effective against what doctors call negative symptoms: having difficulty with day-to-day things and getting on with people. Newer drugs may also help a bit with the thinking problems that people have.

Table 6.4 Drugs against aggression

Drug name	Dose	
Haloperidol	15 mg	Antipsychotic medication can be given with
Olanzapine	10 mg	lorazepam, which is a drug used against
Risperidone	1–2 mg	anxiety.

This is because the newer drugs help increase the amount of dopamine in the thinking part of the brain.

Effects against mood problems

Sometimes people's mood can become elevated or high. Both new and old antipsychotic drugs can help bring people's mood down to a more normal level. Some of the newer antipsychotics also seem to be helpful against low mood or depression that people with psychosis often get.

Effects against aggression

When people have altered experiences, such as feeling paranoid or hearing voices, they can sometimes be so distressed and upset that they become agitated or aggressive. The best way of helping people when they are agitated or distressed is to talk to them. People may need medication to help them with the intense feelings of agitation or aggression they are experiencing. Some antipsychotic drugs (see Table 6.4) are useful in helping people feel calmer. Lorazepam is an anti-anxiety drug that doctors and nurses can also give at the same time as an antipsychotic drug. Some people who have been agitated or aggressive in the past and have found that a particular drug has helped, want to make sure they get the same treatment if these symptoms come back. You can do this by completing an advance directive or crisis card that is described a bit later in this chapter. In England the National Institute for Health and Clinical Excellence (NICE) has published a guideline on the management of violence. If you are interested in reading this guideline you can download a version for the public from their website (www.nice.org.uk).

New (atypical) compared to old (typical) antipsychotics

Most doctors think that new antipsychotic drugs are better than the old ones (see Table 6.5). Clozapine is the most effective antipsychotic drug, but it can only be given to people who have not had any benefit with other

Table 6.5 New compared to old antipsychotic drugs (the higher the score the more effective they are)

Drug name	How good (4 = most effective, 1 = least effective)
Clozapine (only for people who have got no benefit from other antipsychotics)	4
Olanzapine	3
Amisulpiride	3
Risperidone	3
Aripiprazole	2
Quetiapine	2
All old drugs (e.g., haloperidol)	2

antipsychotic drugs because it causes lots of side effects. Of the new antipsychotic drugs, olanzapine, amisulpiride, and risperidone seem to be the most effective. Aripiprazole and quetiapine seem to be as effective as older drugs.

How long do I need to take antipsychotic medication for?

People taking antipsychotic medication often want to know how long they will need to take it for. Doctors and nurses generally advise that people continue taking antipsychotic medication for at least two years after their symptoms have improved. After two years you should talk to your doctor about gradually stopping medication. Some people may need to take medication for longer. If people are taking clozapine they will probably need to take it for at least five years.

Why do I need to keep taking the pills?

You need to keep taking the pills, because if you stop most people find that their psychotic symptoms come back. This may not happen immediately, it may take six months or even a year for them to return. A small number of people who stop medication find that their symptoms never come back. It is impossible to tell whether symptoms will return when someone stops medication, which is why doctors and nurses advise people to keep taking the pills to be on the safe side.

We also think that every time someone has an episode of psychosis this does harm to the brain. So taking medication not only keeps symptoms under control but protects the brain from the damage that psychosis can cause. It is important that people know this and think about it when considering whether they want to stop (or even have a break) from taking antipsychotic medication.

Thinking about the antipsychotic medication you are taking

Let's list the antipsychotic medication you have taken in the past and are taking now. How good is/was your antipsychotic medication at helping with your target symptom (see Exercise 5)?

Exercise 5: Antipsychotic medication taken in the past

Name of drug	How much (mg per day)	Did you take the medication as prescribed?	Why did you stop taking it?	How helpful was this medication at helping with your target symptom? (use the HOW HELPFUL scale below to score this)

How helpful *was* your antipsychotic against your target symptom?

Not helpful	A bit helpful	Helpful	Very helpful
1	2	3	4

What antipsychotic medication are you currently taking?

Name of drug	How much (mg per day)	Do you take the medication as prescribed?	How helpful is this medication at helping with your target symptom? (use the HOW HELPFUL scale below to score this)

How helpful *is* your antipsychotic against your target symptom?

Not helpful	A bit helpful	Helpful	Very helpful
1	2	3	4

Reflections on antipsychotic medication taken in the past

Having completed the exercise above try answering the questions below and consider the advice in the comment boxes.

1. What was the most helpful antipsychotic you have taken?

Comment box

If the most helpful antipsychotic you have taken is not the one you are taking now, would you want to go back to taking the drug you found most helpful? If not, why? (e.g., it was effective, but it had lots of side effects).

---

2. Do you find antipsychotic medication is helpful at treating your target symptoms? YES/NO
   If NO read the comment box below.

Comment box

If you don't think that antipsychotic medication is very helpful in treating your target symptoms you should talk to your doctor about giving clozapine a try. Clozapine can be very helpful if people have not been helped by other antipsychotic drugs.

---

3. Do you accidentally forget to take antipsychotic medication? YES/NO
   If YES read the comment box below.

Comment box

Accidentally forgetting to take medication can put you at risk of your symptoms coming back. If you accidentally forget to take medication you might want to think about a long-acting risperidone injection. Lots of people find that this is a convenient way of taking medication. If you are not keen on an injection here are three simple ways of helping you to remember.
1. Link taking medication to something you always do every day (e.g., cleaning your teeth).
2. Set a daily alarm on your mobile phone to remind you.
3. Talk to your doctor about only having to take medication once a day.

The drugs don't work

A lot of people stop taking antipsychotic medication because they don't feel that it helps against their target symptom (e.g., "hearing voices," "problems getting on with people," or "getting stressed"). About eight out of ten people find that antipsychotic medication helps them. Two out of ten find that medication does not help them with their problems. If this happens it may be helpful to try a drug called clozapine. Clozapine is a very effective antipsychotic drug, but can only be given to people if they have not got any help from other antipsychotics, such as olanzapine or risperidone. The reason that clozapine can only be used for people who have not been helped with other antipsychotics is because in about 1% of people it can cause a lowering of the white blood cells that your body uses to fight infection. This is potentially very dangerous, and as a result people who take clozapine have to have their blood tested regularly. Clozapine can also cause some other difficult to live with side effects that include feeling very tired, putting on weight, and dribbling. Many people who take clozapine say that it is the best medication they have ever taken and that it really helps them.

Hilary: switching to clozapine

Hilary had heard voices for over ten years. She found them terrifying and distressing. Over the years she had become increasingly more withdrawn and isolated, rarely going out and spending most of her time in her bedroom at her parents' house. She had tried several different antipsychotic medicines including risperidone and amisulpiride, but they had not really helped at all. Although initially reluctant to try clozapine because of the side effects she eventually decided to give it a go. Although clozapine made her very tired and she struggled to get out of bed before midday it really helped with the voices. Although they didn't go away they were not as intense and she was more able to ignore them.

What do people think about taking antipsychotic medication?

Most people who take antipsychotic medication say that there are some positive things about taking medication as well as negatives (see Table 6.6). Very few people think that medication is either all good or all bad. People have to weigh up in their own mind whether – on balance – medication is useful. This can change from day to day. On one day you can think that medication is helpful, on the next you can have had enough of it and want to stop. Listed below in Table 6.6 are some of the things people often say are the good and the not so good things about taking antipsychotic medication.

What do people think about stopping antipsychotic medication?

People not only think about the pros and cons of taking antipsychotic medication, they also think about the pros and cons of stopping medication. Listed in Table 6.7 are some of the pros and cons of stopping medication.

Making the right choice (before you start taking antipsychotic medication)

We have talked a lot about different antipsychotic medications, how they work, what symptoms they help with, and what side effects they cause. Before you start taking antipsychotic medication it can be helpful to weigh up the pros

Table 6.6 The cons and pros of taking antipsychotic medication

Cons	Pros
• Side effects of medication • Worries about taking medication for a long time • Medication not helping with target symptom • It's uncomfortable taking medication (e.g., I find it hard to swallow the tablet; the injection is painful)	• Helps with symptoms • Being able to get on with life • Improvements in relationships • Feeling safe

Table 6.7 The pros and cons of stopping antipsychotic medication

Pros	Cons
• Getting rid of side effects • No stigma of taking medication • Increased autonomy • Not being controlled by medication anymore	• Symptoms getting worse • Going back into hospital • Losing the positive things in life • Losing the calmness

and cons of each medication choice. We have described a decision-making exercise (see Exercise 7) that may help you think about how each choice may affect you.

Do I keep taking the pills?

People who are taking antipsychotic medication are often unsure about whether they want to keep taking it. People's view about whether medication is *important* or not change from day to day. There are six main factors that affect how important people think antipsychotic medication is. These factors are as follows.

- Does medication help with my target symptoms?
- Am I aware of how to manage the side effects I can get from my medication?
- Do I have a good relationship with the mental health professional that looks after me?
- Do the side effects that I get bother me?
- Has medication helped me in the past?
- Do I believe that medication helps with my problems?

Reflection

What do you think about antipsychotic medication? Do you think it is important? Take five minutes to reflect on what you think about antipsychotic medication. Then complete Exercise 6.

Exercise 6

Is medication important?

How important do you think it is to keep taking the pills?

1 2 3 4 5 6 7 8 9 10
←Not important   Very important→

Why did you place yourself at that particular point on the scale?

What would have to happen for medication to become more important?

What can you do to address this problem?

George: "keep taking the pills"

George had been taking olanzapine for about six months. It had helped him cope with the voices he hears, but he had put on weight and really felt that he should not rely on medication as a "crutch." George rated medication as five out of ten on the importance scale. He felt that although he didn't like relying on medication, at this point in his life he needed it to cope. The main problem with his olanzapine was that he had put on weight. George felt that he wanted help to try and lose the weight he had put on. He met with his nurse and used the problem-solving template on page 122 to work out ways of losing weight.

Key message

There are often practical problems that people have with medication. You and the mental health professional that works with you can make use of the problem-solving template on page 122 to find your own solutions.

It is natural to think about stopping taking medication. Perhaps you will wake up one morning and think "I don't need medication any more, I am fine and I can cope on my own." In a similar way to choosing to take medication by considering the pros and cons of each medication choice, it is important to think carefully about whether you keep on taking it. You may want to think again about the pros and cons of taking and stopping anti-psychotic medication. Is it right for you? What problems do you have with medication? Do you need to think about changing to a different medication?

Key message

If you ever decide that you want to stop medication always do this gradually working with your doctor or nurse. Never stop medication suddenly, as this can make you feel restless, agitated, and cause sleeping problems. This happens because it takes time for your body to adjust to stopping medication.

Exercise 7

Weighing up the pros and cons can be helpful. If you are taking antipsychotic medication why not complete Exercise 7.

Write the name of the medication you are taking in the first box, and then fill in the four boxes:
- The helpful things about taking medication
- The unhelpful things about taking medication
- The helpful things about stopping medication
- The unhelpful things about stopping medication.

What is the name of the medication:	
If I take/keep taking this medication . . .	
The helpful things about taking medication (list your thoughts below)	The unhelpful things about taking medication (list your thoughts below)
If I stop/don't take my medication . . .	
The helpful things about stopping medication (list your thoughts below)	The unhelpful things about stopping medication (list your thoughts below)

Think about your answers. Where does that leave you now? Is this medication right for you?

Completing this exercise can often throw up lots of practical problems, especially about the side effects of antipsychotic medication. Side effects of medication are dealt with next.

A rough guide to the side effects of antipsychotic medications

No medication is side effect free and antipsychotic drugs are no different. They can cause a number of side effects that can be unpleasant and difficult to live with.

Side effects tend to be more common:
- when starting antipsychotic medication
- when the dose of medication is high

- when the dose of medication is increased
- in children
- in people over the age of 65 (older adults).

Exercise 8 should help you work out what side effects you are getting from medication and think about which ones are more distressing (harder to live with).

Exercise 8

Identifying side effects

Part one: List the side effects you are currently experiencing from your antipsychotic medication (just write them down as they come to mind, don't worry about the order they are in):

Part two: Now that you have listed the side effects you are getting, we need to put them into some kind of order. Take a few minutes to look at the list you have written and think about which of the side effects you find most distressing and which less distressing. Give each side effect a distress score out of 10 (10 = most distressing to 1 = not distressing at all).

Side effect distress score

1   2   3   4   5   6   7   8   9   10
←Least distressing   Most distressing→

Now that you have given each side effect a score, list the side effects that you find most distressing here:

The side effects I find most distressing are:

1.

2.

3.

These are the side effects that you should try and get some help sorting out. Remember you should not have to suffer in silence; most of the time something can be done to help you.

Before we discuss what you can do to manage side effects it is helpful to look at some of the common side effects that antipsychotics can cause. These include:

- movement problems – including stiffness, shakiness, restlessness, and strange unusual movements
- period problems in women
- breast enlargement (in men and women)
- sexual dysfunction
- fits (especially with high doses of medication and with clozapine)
- low blood pressure
- dry mouth
- blurred vision
- constipation
- weight gain
- feeling very tired.

Sorting out side effects

There are different ways of trying to get rid of the side effects of antipsychotic medication. Sometimes reducing the amount of medication you take each day or changing the time of day that you take it can get rid of side effects (for example if your medication makes you feel tired it is better to take it at night rather than in the morning so you are not sleepy during the day). Other ways of helping with side effects include:

- changing the medication you are taking from one antipsychotic to another, for example, if you a getting movement problems
- giving you another drug, such as a laxative, if you are constipated and you are having difficulty going to the toilet
- making lifestyle changes, such as eating a more healthy diet and exercising more, if medication makes you put on weight.

We have listed ways of helping with some of the common side effects from antipsychotic medication in Table 6.8.

To sort out some of the side effects you get from antipsychotic medication you may need to work with your doctor or nurse. We have found that it can often be very helpful to try and work through problems in a structured way. This is the best way of finding a solution to a problem that suits you. A problem-solving process might look something like this:

- What is the problem?
- What is the goal?
- When do you aim to achieve your goal (date)?
- What are the different ways of achieving this goal?

Table 6.8 Ways of sorting out side effects

Side effect	What can be done
• Movement problems – including stiffness, shakiness, restlessness, and strange unusual movements	• Reduce the amount of medication prescribed • Give an antidote e.g., procyclidine • Change the medication
• Period problems in women	• Reduce the amount of medication prescribed • Change the medication
• Breast enlargement (in men and women)	• Reduce the amount of medication prescribed • Change the medication
• Sexual dysfunction	• Reduce the amount of medication prescribed • Change the medication
• Fits (especially with high doses of medication and with clozapine)	• Reduce the amount of medication prescribed • Possibly give a drug against fits
• Low blood pressure	• Start with a small amount of medication and gradually increase the dose • Get out of bed/stand up slowly
• Dry mouth	• Change the medication • Sip lots of water (not pop/fizzy drinks) • Chew sugar free chewing gum
• Blurred vision	• Change the medication
• Constipation	• Change the medication • Take a laxative • Eat a high fiber diet • Exercise
• Putting on weight	• Change medication • Diet changes • Increase daily activity/exercise
• Feeling very tired	• Take medication before bed rather than first thing in the morning

- What are the pros and cons of each way of achieving this goal?
- What is the best way of achieving this goal for me?
- What are the barriers that might get in the way of achieving this goal?
- What needs to be in an action plan for achieving your goal?
- Have you achieved your goal?

Let's look at an example of how problem solving might work in practice.

Kathy: "I want to lose weight"

Kathy had been taking olanzapine for four months and had put on three stones in weight.

What is the problem?

Kathy said that the problem was: "I have gained three stones in weight since I started taking the medication. This makes me feel self-conscious and I don't like going out."

What is the goal?

Initially Kathy said she wanted to "lose weight" but her nurse suggested that this needed to be "more specific." So they agreed that the goal should be to lose 6 lbs in three months.

What are the different ways of achieving this goal?

Kathy and her nurse identified five ways of achieving this goal. They were:

1. Eat very little
2. Change what I eat
3. Exercise
4. Reduce the medication
5. Stop the medication.

What are the pros and cons of each way of solving this problem?

Kathy said she felt too hungry to reduce what she ate. She also said that she didn't know what the healthy foods she should be eating were. She said "I don't like exercising and cannot afford to go to a gym" and that "sometimes I feel OK when I reduce the medication, though when I have stopped it for long periods I get ill again."

What is the best way of achieving this goal for me?

Kathy decided that for her the best way of achieving her goal was to try and find out more about healthy foods and try and avoid sugary and fatty foods that she thought made her fat.

What are the barriers that might get in the way of achieving this goal?

Kathy thought that the main barrier to achieving her goal was about how to find out information.

What needs to be in an action plan for achieving this goal?

Kathy said she would get a book out from the library that "will tell me about healthy food." Her nurse also said that she would bring some leaflets about healthy foods.

Kathy said she wanted to make a plan of the foods she might eat more of and foods she might eat less of.

A "healthy eating start date" was agreed.

(Continued)

They agreed that Kathy would weigh herself on the scales in her bathroom every week on a Sunday evening and keep a weight loss diary.

The nurse who was working with Kathy said she would phone her twice a week just to check how she was getting on with the diet.

Have you achieved your goal?

After three months Kathy had been successful in working out a healthy eating plan and set a healthy eating start date. Kathy managed to change her diet but over the three-month period had had a couple of "lapses" when she had a "junk food binge." She weighed herself every week and kept a diary. After three months she had lost four pounds. Kathy particularly valued the positive feedback she had had from her nurse when she phoned. Kathy said "my nurse was always positive even when I lapsed, that kept me going."

Exercise 9 is a problem-solving template. You can fill it in on your own, with the help of someone in your family, or with the health care professional working with you.

Exercise 9

Problem solving

What is the problem?

What is the goal?

What are the different ways of achieving this goal?

What are the pros and cons of each way of solving this problem?

What is the best way of achieving this goal for me?

What are the barriers that might get in the way of achieving this goal?

What needs to be in an action plan for achieving this goal?

Have you achieved your goal?

Key message

All antipsychotic drugs can cause side effects. Something can be done about any side effect that occurs. Do not suffer in silence – talk to your doctor or nurse.

Making choices about medication in advance

For lots of reasons people's mental health symptoms can get worse and they find it difficult to cope. Often when these mental health crises happen professionals have to respond to them. Many people with mental health problems are unhappy about how they are treated when crises occur. This is often because choices are made for them by carers or mental health workers. For example, a person may be prescribed a medication they don't like by a doctor they don't know. This can be avoided. You can make choices about what you want to happen if a mental health crisis occurs. Sometimes people call this an "advance direction" or "crisis plan." Exercise 10 is an example of a crisis plan that you might want to use.

Exercise 10

Making medication choices in advance

Below is an example of a crisis plan that you can complete either on your own or with your mental health worker. It may be helpful to give a copy of the crisis plan to your psychiatrist, your family, and your mental health worker.

Exercise 10 (Continued)

Name:

Address:

Date:

1. If I have a mental health crisis this is how I usually feel . . .

2. The medication/treatment that I want is (think about dose, how it is administered (e.g., tablet/injection), how often you take it) . . .

3. The medication/treatment I DO NOT want is (or way of taking medication e.g., injection) . . .

4. The reasons for this is . . .

If I am agitated or aggressive it helps me if . . .

I would like the people looking after me to know the following (think about what you like to eat, any physical health problems you may have, any religious customs, any practical issues e.g., who will feed the cat/pay bills) . . .

I would like the following people to be contacted . . .

I would like the following people to look after my children/dependants (if applicable) . . .

Signature:

Date:

Signature of witness:

Date:

> ### A final thought: putting medication in its place
>
> Antipsychotic medication can be an important part of helping you manage your symptoms and helping you recover from a psychosis. But it is just part of a package of care and treatment that may include psychological support, social care, and lifelong education and training. Prescribed carefully and managed well, medication should not get in the way of you achieving your life goals. Antipsychotic medication should help you to achieve them.

Cultural and religious aspects

In certain cultures medication is not the treatment of choice for psychosis, and people prefer exorcists or local healers to treat them. There is nothing wrong with following your cultural traditions, as long as you have explored all options including medication. It may be that you choose to try both together. Although cultural traditions date back many years, research into medical treatments has also been extensive over the years.

If English is not your first language, you can ask for information about your medication in a different language. This is very important, as until you understand what the medication is about you will not feel the need to take it. You need to be involved in the choice of medication and your overall treatment plan. If need be discuss this with a professional from your own background.

Summary

If you don't want to read the whole of this interesting and useful chapter, here are eight key points for you to think about.

1. Talking to your health care professional can be difficult. Work out what you want to ask in advance and make sure you get answers to your questions.
2. Psychosis affects different people in different ways. Work out for yourself what the target problem is that you need help with.
3. There are different types of antipsychotic medication. Some are more effective than others.
4. All antipsychotic medications can cause side effects. If you get side effects don't suffer in silence – get help.

5. You need to choose which antipsychotic medication best suits you.
6. If you stop taking medication there is a good chance your psychotic symptoms will come back.
7. If symptoms come back, plan in advance what medication you want.
8. Antipsychotic medication should enable you to achieve your life goals.

Why me? Why now? Understanding vulnerability from a cognitive perspective

Alison Brabban

Overview

This chapter aims to offer the reader an understanding of how negative attitudes (schemas) can work to keep psychotic symptoms going and prevent recovery. Techniques are described to identify such schemas and to develop more positive attitudes.

Chapter contents

- The stress vulnerability model
- Core beliefs or schema
- Early events and the development of schema
- Cognitive distortions
- Conditional beliefs
- Timelines: exploring schema-defining events
- Improving negative schemas

If you have had psychotic-type experiences such as hearing voices or feeling paranoid, you may well be asking yourself "why has this happened to me?" and "why now?" Throughout the book, a number of the chapters have referred to the stress vulnerability model as a way of making sense of why someone can experience psychotic symptoms. Different people use different metaphors to explain this model including Sarah Wilcock who in Chapter 8 uses the analogy of a pan of water boiling over to describe it. The emphasis of this metaphor is on the "stress" element of the stress vulnerability model. Of course, not everyone who gets stressed out or who has to deal with traumatic events in their lives has psychotic experiences, so why do some people experience psychosis and not others?

The fact of the matter is that no one knows the answer to this question for certain, so it is impossible to predict who will and who will not become psychotic. However, we do know that some things can contribute to increasing the likelihood that a person may experience psychosis. Let's go back to the stress vulnerability model again and focus on the vulnerability aspect of the model. This time we're going to think about the model using a bucket filling with water to explain it.

The stress vulnerability model

It appears that most people if not everyone has some level of vulnerability to developing psychotic symptoms: while some people are highly vulnerable, others seem to have merely a minimal susceptibility. Using a bucket analogy, vulnerability is represented by the bucket. People who are extremely vulnerable can be thought of as small buckets and not able to deal with much water/stress going in before the bucket overflows; whereas those people who have minimal vulnerability can be compared to very large buckets with plenty of room to cope with lots of water/stress.

The size of the bucket, in other words the level of vulnerability, is determined by a lot of different factors. Genes play a part, which means that people who have blood relatives that have experienced psychotic symptoms or mental health problems may be more vulnerable to developing problems themselves. Genes are only one part of the picture, however; genes interact with a number of other factors to determine overall vulnerability. Our childhood, where we lived, things that happened to us, and relationships we had, all can play a part. For example, we know that certain unpleasant experiences during childhood including things such as bullying, abuse, or being placed in care can all increase the likelihood of developing psychotic experiences later in life. Social factors also play a part, and it seems that even growing up in an inner city or built-up area, or as part of a disadvantaged minority ethnic group, might make a person more vulnerable (i.e., it might make the bucket smaller). These different biological, psychological, and social elements come together to determine not only the *type* of stressors we find most difficult to deal with, but what happens to us when the stress gets too much.

As previous chapters have said, our level of vulnerability is only one factor in explaining why people experience psychotic symptoms; stress also seems to play a part. In the stress vulnerability model, stress is compared to water coming into the bucket. If a lot of water comes into the bucket, in other words if a person experiences a great deal of personal stress, then the bucket can overflow, which is when psychotic symptoms can occur. People who have a low level of vulnerability can be compared to "big buckets" that are able to cope with more stress (water) than those who have a high level of vulnerability – the equivalent of a small bucket. Stress comes in lots of forms: losing a job, a relationship split, bereavements, being assaulted, financial problems, housing problems – the list is endless. Sometimes things that people see as exciting can still cause a lot of stress, such as getting married, leaving home, or going on holiday.

Finally, certain things make it more or less likely that the bucket will overflow. This can be thought of as akin to holes in the bottom of the bucket. The holes are like a plughole in a bath. As long as the plughole is unblocked and the water isn't pouring in too fast, then the bath won't overflow. However, if the plughole gets blocked then it is much more likely that if the tap is running, even slowly, then a flood will ensue. The holes in the bottom of the bucket allow most of us to cope with the everyday stresses and strains of day-to-day life without it overflowing or the stress getting too much. Unfortunately, some things have the effect of "blocking the holes" while other things seem to "clear the holes." The holes in the bottom of the bucket are the equivalent of good and bad coping strategies. Probably the most common thing that has the impact of blocking the holes and making it likely that the bucket will overflow is lack of sleep. Most people who are sufficiently sleep deprived will experience psychotic symptoms. Certain drugs such as amphetamine and cannabis can also have the effect of "blocking the holes." However, just as some things can make it more likely that the bucket will overflow, so some things open the holes and seem to help us cope with the stress: medication, sharing problems, relaxation, and writing down feelings are examples of things that might help.

So if the stress/water exceeds the capacity of a person to cope/the size of the bucket and it overflows, then a person might experience psychotic symptoms such as hearing voices, seeing things, or getting quite mixed up in their thinking. How then do we explain why for some people these symptoms aren't a temporary thing, but last for a long time? Well, if someone has a very high vulnerability then even the general stress of living will be enough to keep the bucket overflowing. Also, once a person starts experiencing strange psychotic-type experiences then these in themselves cause a lot of stress for the person and can keep the bucket spilling over. However, by reducing the stress sufficiently or by helping the person to cope with the stress in their life (opening the holes in the bucket), then the bucket will stop overflowing and the psychotic experiences will diminish or disappear altogether.

Core beliefs or schema

The stress vulnerability model is a simple, helpful way to understand how biological, social, and psychological factors all can play a part in the development of mental health problems, whether this is psychosis or not. For some people, an excess of stress may lead to anxiety problems or depression rather than psychotic experiences. This is all determined by your "make up": those biological, psychological, and social factors that make up the size and shape of your bucket and the holes that are there. We can take the stress vulnerability model to a deeper level of understanding, however, to appreciate why events in our childhood might make us more sensitive or vulnerable to certain events later in life.

Have you noticed that certain events make you more anxious than others? You might be fine going fast on a motor bike yet be terrified of walking into a room full of strangers; alternatively, social situations might not be a problem for you at all but you would be panicked if you had to sit an exam or be tested in some way. Most of us have particular areas in our lives that we find more difficult to deal with than others. We might worry about these if we are confronted with them, or we might choose to avoid them altogether so that we don't have to deal with a heightened level of stress. The cognitive therapy model as described by Aaron T. Beck provides some clues to help us understand why this might be.

The model suggests that the way we think about ourselves and the world is colored by certain "core beliefs" that we hold about ourselves and others. Beck called these core beliefs "schema." Core beliefs or schema are seen as important elements of the cognitive model as they can color or distort the way we see ourselves and our world. So where do our schema come from? Schema are fundamentally the result of us trying to make sense of our lives. From birth we are confronted with new situations on a daily basis, which we try to make sense of and understand. Understanding how things work and being able to make predictions is a necessary aspect of human life. Babies will learn through countless "experiments" the impact their actions have on others around them and on their environment. This in turn leads to the development of intentional actions based on the realization that their actions make a difference. As an example, they may learn that pushing a food bowl at arm's length makes it disappear over the edge of the table, or that if they squash their toy rabbit it squeaks, and so on. As children grow older so their level of understanding becomes more sophisticated.

Early events and the development of schema

Making sense of our world is an essential survival strategy. Through both positive and negative experiences we learn what is safe and what is dangerous and to be avoided. Putting our hand in the fire is painful and to be avoided, whereas smiling at grandma results in a cuddle. This learning and understanding helps us predict how things work and how others are likely to respond to us: it helps us deal with the challenges of day-to-day life and shapes the way we behave. When faced with totally new experiences, or events that don't follow predicted patterns, then we will often feel out of sorts or anxious. Schema are the core beliefs about ourselves, other people, and about the world that we have developed from our experiences during our childhood. They guide us to predict what will happen in the different situations that we face. So, for example, if someone felt mainly cared for and loved while he was growing up, it is likely that he will have a healthy level of self-esteem. His core belief about himself might be "I am good enough as I am" and about others might be "other people are kind and considerate." As a result he will face situations with confidence, expecting that others will treat him with respect. On the other hand, if a child were constantly bullied by his peers and told by his family that he was "a waste of space" then it is more likely that this person would have made sense of his life more negatively. His core beliefs about himself might be "I'm unlovable." He might also think that "other people are cruel and will reject me." Unlike the person in the first example, this man is more likely to be wary of other people and be quite anxious in social situations.

Examples of types of behavior that people might be exposed to and associated core beliefs they might develop

Constant criticism	=	"There's something wrong with me"
Mollycoddled/overprotected	=	"I'm vulnerable and need protecting"
Shown no love or affection	=	"I can never get enough love"
Spoilt	=	"I am entitled to whatever I want"

As well as learning from our own experiences, we often adopt the values, beliefs, and opinions of those around us. For example, if religion played a significant part in your upbringing then it is likely that your beliefs will be influenced by the religious teachings you heard and lived with. Each different cultural group, be it working class or middle class, southerner or northerner, Indian or African, Tory or Socialist, Jew or Muslim, goth or hippie, 60s child or 90s child, will have its own related values and core beliefs. Our own personal core beliefs will therefore be influenced by the different cultural groups we grew up with and who we identify with.

Childhood events

(including cultural norms, significant relationships, positive experiences, early adversity, etc.)

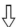

Core beliefs about ourselves, other people, and the world such as
"I am ... "
"The world is ... "
"Other people are ... "

Core beliefs might be helpful in some ways, in that they allow us to feel that we understand the world and can predict what is going to happen. Unfortunately, they can also lead to problems. When we develop a core belief then this can color and actually distort the way we make sense of our lives on a day-to-day basis.

Every day we are faced with lots of ambiguous situations, situations that are not completely clear cut in terms of understanding what is going on, and we will try to make sense of these. We might not be offered a job that we felt we were qualified to do; someone might look at us in a peculiar way while we are out; a neighbor who you know well might not acknowledge you when you pass her in the street. In each of these situations and situations like them, we will attempt to understand why this happened. Unfortunately, this is where our core beliefs can get in the way. When we try and work out what was going on we use our understanding of ourselves, other people, and the world to help us – and this can bias our conclusions.

Let's take the above example of the neighbor not acknowledging us in the street. There are many different reasons why this might have happened. She might have not seen us; she might have had a lot on her mind and she was distracted; she might have had a row with her husband and not wanted to speak to anyone; she might have decided she doesn't want anything to do with us anymore. The list is endless. Nevertheless, as I said earlier, we all want to make some sense of our world so the chances are we will try to work out why our neighbor isn't acknowledging us today. This is where our schema come in: we are more likely to make sense of current situations in light of previous experiences. So even though two people (let's say Peter and Paul, for the example) are confronted with exactly the same situation, they might come up with different explanations. If Peter has experiences of people as unreliable and rejecting then he will be much more likely to decide that his neighbor is also unreliable and rejecting and doesn't want anything to do with him anymore. Paul, on the other hand, might always have been very popular and not had any negative experiences of rejection. He is more likely to believe that the neighbor is evidently distracted or has not seen him and this was not a personal slight.

Cognitive distortions

What we know about this process of making sense of our lives is that we are all biased in our judgments. Our schema or core beliefs lead us to sometimes distort the information that is available to us. We are more likely to focus on aspects of the situation that fit with our beliefs and discount the bits that don't tally with what we believe. However, sometimes we are faced with heaps of evidence that doesn't fit with our core beliefs. When this happens this state of "not knowing" can make us uncomfortable. Let's take the example of Peter above, who has had bad experiences of other people. His belief is that "people are unkind and not to be trusted." If he is confronted with someone who is kind, considerate, and seems genuinely concerned, it will be difficult for him to fit this new behavior into his core belief system. He won't quite know how to make sense of this person's apparent kindness because, after all, his belief is that "people are unkind."

When faced with situations where there is a mismatch between our current lives and events in our past that shaped our core beliefs, we have two options open to us to reduce the discomfort of not knowing that this brings. The first is to change our core beliefs to fit the new situation, or alternatively we can actually distort the way we perceive the current situation so that it matches our beliefs. In the case of Peter, if he were to change his core belief or schema, it might change from "people *generally* are unkind and not to be trusted" to "*some* people are unkind and not to be trusted." Alternatively, if he were to go down the second route, he could reduce the discomfort by distorting his perception of what he observed. He could minimize the significance of meeting someone so benevolent by thinking "yes he was kind-hearted, but he's one in a million" or he could discount the other person's behavior altogether by concluding "that wasn't genuine kindness." These distortions allow us to keep our core beliefs intact and let us feel as though we have ourselves and the world sussed, thereby reducing the discomfort of not knowing.

Cognitive therapists recognize a number of types of "cognitive distortions" that keep core beliefs from being challenged. Some of these are listed in Table 7.1.

So far I have talked about how events in our childhood lead us to understand ourselves and others in particular ways. These core beliefs become the spectacles by which we view our worlds. If we have had a particularly good, secure upbringing, then these spectacles might be rose tinted, but they can also become muddied by adversity and suffering. It seems our core beliefs play an important role in helping us understand events in the world. They also play a significant role in determining how we behave.

Conditional beliefs

As humans, if we believe there is a problem then we have a tendency to try to rectify this in some way. So, if dad is always telling you that you are a waste of space, and you conclude that you aren't good enough (your schema), then you may decide to do something that will *make* you good enough. If dad is a successful business man, then you may decide that if you work hard and are a success then you might achieve "good enough" status. We know that people often develop certain "rules for living" that will overcome or compensate for

Table 7.1 Examples of cognitive distortions

Black and white thinking	Things are seen as all or nothing, e.g., unless it was perfect then it was a complete waste of time.
Over-generalization	The significance of an event is exaggerated, e.g., a teacher who has a single bad lesson, concludes they're a useless teacher and should give up on their chosen career.
Mental filter	One small aspect of a much bigger situation is focused on at the expense of everything else, e.g., one bad mark is focused on, even though the person got nine other extremely good marks.
Jumping to conclusions	A person decides what is going on without taking all of the facts into consideration, e.g., a friend doesn't call when they said they would and this is interpreted as "she doesn't like me" when there are lots of other potential explanations.
Emotional reasoning	Reasoning is based on feelings rather than facts, e.g., "I feel like people are out to get me so it must be true."

their own perceived flaws. These rules are what cognitive therapists call "conditional beliefs" or "assumptions." They tend to present in the form of "if . . . then . . . " statements such as in the example above. These conditional beliefs often drive us to behave in certain ways or patterns in order to make things better.

As an example, Jenny's life became difficult at the age of eight when her family moved up to the north of England from the south. She started a new school and found it difficult to fit in. It seemed that everyone was making fun of her and her "posh southern accent." To make matters worse around the same age she had to start wearing a brace on her teeth, and this gave her peers further ammunition to tease her and make her life pretty miserable. This went on for months and she started to believe "there's something wrong with me, I don't fit in" (a core belief or schema). To try and make herself more popular she developed a plan, she would always try to be pleasant to everyone and try not to upset anyone in any way. If she could help someone in any way then she would, even if this involved doing something she didn't particularly enjoy. She developed the conditional belief "If I try and please people then they might accept me." The good news for Jenny was that this seemed to work for her, people did seem to want her around. Others commented that she always seemed to be "smiley and happy," unfortunately, Jenny didn't always feel like this inside. More and more she started to feel taken advantage of and yet she never felt she could show any anger or irritation; she was worried that if she didn't always please people they would reject her again. A problem for Jenny was that her self-esteem was pretty low, and she didn't truly believe that people liked her for who she was. She had to be pleasant and happy at all times, even if she felt angry or sad, or people wouldn't want her around. The other issue was that if she felt that someone wasn't particularly keen on her, then she would work even harder to get them to like her. At these times she would be even kinder or be even more giving, whatever the response was she got back. Sometimes she found that people took advantage of her kindness, but she felt unable to assert herself. So although Jenny's conditional belief had helped her to some extent in that she now had some friends, it also had its disadvantages as she felt that people didn't accept her for who she was and she found that people took advantage of her. Overall, Jenny's core beliefs and conditional beliefs made her more anxious about relationships and about social situations. Any kind of rejection or situation that resonated with her childhood experiences hit her hard. She always blamed herself and triggered her core belief that she "wasn't good enough."

Going back to the stress vulnerability model, we can view our childhood experiences, and the way they shaped our beliefs about ourselves, the world, and other people, as determining our own individual vulnerabilities. People who were bullied or victimized as children may find it more stressful if they are confronted with events later in life that mirror some elements of these early experiences than others who have not had these same childhood experiences. Similarly, if a little girl was "overprotected," and started to believe that she "needed looking after," then for her being alone later in life would be a particularly difficult situation to deal with. Going back to the bucket analogy, our bucket (own personal vulnerability) is formed not only by our biological make up but by our early experiences and core beliefs. Our childhood experiences and the resulting schema determine the types of event that we will find particularly stressful later in life: they can be thought of as our psychological Achilles heel.

Although a cognitive therapist can work to help people change their unhealthy schema, it is beyond the scope of this book to look at how this is done. It might be helpful, however, to understand which events in your earlier life might have contributed to your own vulnerability. These events might provide a clue to your own core beliefs about you, the world, and other people.

Timelines: exploring schema-defining events

Timelines were introduced in Chapter one as a way of helping you reflect on what might trigger a psychotic episode. To help explore the events that have led to your own psychological vulnerabilities, try doing another timeline, but this time extend it back to your birth and continue it right the way through to the present day. Add all the major events in your life that spring to mind. These might include starting different schools, any bereavements or losses, moving house, particular outstandingly happy times such as a family holiday or a sporting achievement, and times that were memorably unhappy. Don't worry if you can't remember much the first time round, write down what you *can* remember and you can revisit your timeline again later and add things that have come to mind. When people complete a timeline they are often surprised how much they have had to deal with in their lives. Many people who have had psychotic experiences have had to deal with more than their fair share of adversity during their lives. Once your timeline has a few events on it, you will be able to reflect on your own life. If you want you can also think about *what you made* of these events at the time they happened. For an example you might have failed an exam and believed "I'm stupid"; you might have been beaten on a regular basis and in the eyes of a child you might have thought "this is my fault." Reflecting on the significant events and relationships in your life might help you consider what might constitute your own personal psychological vulnerabilities.

Improving negative schemas

By examining the life events that you were dealing with prior to your psychosis, you may see that you were dealing with similar issues and feelings that caused you difficulties in the past. If this makes you think that there are significant parts of your life that you feel you have not dealt with before and that you know or suspect are causing problems for you now, then talk to your primary care physician or mental health worker (if you have one) about being referred to a therapist who can help you explore and deal with these issues. Alternatively, Jeffrey Young and Janet Klosko have written a self-help book to help people identify and deal with their own core beliefs and to overcome the negative life patterns that these beliefs promote. One simple way of improving negative schemas is to practice bringing to mind positive memories and feelings from your past. Initially these might be difficult to think of, as voices and paranoia can take up so much of your thinking time. People with psychosis sometimes come to believe that they have failed in life. An antidote to this negative attitude might be to remember once a day for ten minutes a couple of times in your life when you definitely succeeded. Examples might include scoring a winning goal for the school football or hockey team, or an example of a close friendship, or a period of successful study. Write down below three definite success experiences from earlier in your life, and also write how you felt at the time.

1.

2.

3.

Now practice really remembering and developing these memories and getting in touch with those pleasant feelings of achievement. By practicing this any negative attitudes you might have about failure will begin to be less powerful.

FURTHER READING

Young, J. E. & Klosko, J. S. (1998). *Reinventing your Life: How to Break Free from Negative Life Patterns.* USA: Penguin Putnam Inc.

8

Helping carers help themselves using a cognitive approach

Sarah K. J. Wilcock

Overview

This chapter aims to offer the reader an understanding of how carers can use cognitive therapy to help themselves to cope better and then to become an active participant in their psychotic relative's or friend's recovery.

Chapter contents

- What is a carer?
- Role of the carer
- Expressed emotion
- Case studies
- Stress
- Stress management
- Cognitive approach to self-help
- Cultural and religious aspects
- Summary

Caring is by no means an easy role. I took on the role as carer for my grandmother in my late teens, following the death of my father. Originally the role involved a visit every Saturday, occasionally purchasing her groceries or collecting her money. However, as time moved on and she became more frail, my duties became more substantive. Purchasing my grandmother's groceries did not seem too much of a challenge at first, even though she could only eat certain foods that had to be ordered. She was also very particular with respect to the size of her potatoes! However, for food that I had to order, it had to be picked up from the store three or four times a week and delivered to her that same day. At this time, I was working approximately ten miles away from both the store and my grandmother, hence when the task had to be undertaken three or four times a week I started to feel under pressure. On these days I would leave work in my lunch break, drive to the local town, try and park the car, retrieve the goods as quickly as possible from the store, drop the groceries off, and rush back to work. I followed this routine for a couple of years before going to university. University was a lot further away than my employer, and due to the nature of my course and placements involved it meant that I was much less flexible than before. While studying full time, I also maintained a job part time (22 hours per week). This was when I really felt under pressure, and stressed by my responsibilities. For the next three years I juggled my time, studying and work, around purchasing my grandmother's groceries, and relied on close friends and my partner to help me out. Throughout this time I experienced varying emotions depending on how I was feeling in myself and what was happening around me, e.g., personal relationships, employment, and course work for my studies.

I recall on numerous occasions simply running into the house with the goods and running out again, not realizing how that made her feel, i.e., a burden on me. One day when I did have time and stayed longer to talk to her, she asked me why I was making conversation, as a result I felt so guilty. Other emotions I experienced were sheer frustration with my circumstance, distress, and, at times when I was unsure as to how I would manage, resentment towards her, as a result of not being able to cope. I also recall a day when she left a message on my answer machine repeating the words "food, food, food – what am I going to do?" My response was that of rage and anger. I'd reached my breaking point. I picked up the answer machine, threw it down the hall, and cried for some time afterwards. Although I acknowledge that my experience of a caring role was not for an individual suffering from a severe mental illness, the experience of the actual responsibility opened my eyes to the pressure and stress involved. There was also stress as a result of the array of negative feelings and emotions evoked, which clearly had an impact on me and my life. My role continued for approximately nine years until my grandmother passed away at the grand age of 91. On reflection I'm surprised I managed to cope as long as I did, without any support from social services throughout these years. I was unaware of what services were available to me, but also reluctant to attempt to access them due to how set in her ways my grandmother was. I also believe that due to my age, I was not recognized as a carer but a grand-daughter fulfilling her role within the family.

Since this time I have watched others around me experience similar difficulties, e.g., my mother caring for my step-father, again with limited support. I support her to the best of my ability; however, now I tend to focus on her mental health needs within her role, more so than practical support, with a view to helping her help herself.

What is a carer?

There is often a misunderstanding as to who exactly constitutes a carer. A "carer" is not only a person being paid to undertake a caring role or a volunteer within the caring field, but can also be a concerned or devoted individual who is reliable or supportive towards a sufferer of an illness. Carers can be recognized as young or old and can be any member of the family, e.g., mum or dad, son or daughter, siblings, grandchild, or a friend, or even a neighbor. A carer is simply anyone who provides substantial care on a regular basis (DoH, 2002, PDS, 2003).

Following the 2001 census, the government recognized that there were approximately 6.8 million carers in England. Further monitoring highlighted that 1.5 million of these were carers for individuals suffering a mental illness (DoH, 2006). Carers fill a key role and provide invaluable support to individual sufferers or "service users," often in the long term, and are seldom aware of the depth of their responsibility and commitment. A role or responsibility of this nature brings with it a vast array of positive and negative experiences for both the carer and the service user, therefore one ought not be surprised or offended if you were to hear terms such as "burden of care" or "difficulty coping." Once established within the role of a carer, a person may begin to notice the impact of such responsibility on themselves and the service user both physically and mentally. Furthermore, one may also begin to observe how the service user's reactions to such support and level of functioning or independence may change for the better or the worse. In turn, depending on the outcome of such support, this can have a massive impact on the carer's role and responsibilities, now and in the future.

The role of the carer has always been apparent and appreciated, but not necessarily from a statutory perspective, although in recent years the role has become increasingly recognized and valued by support services and the government, who have now acknowledged this in recent government proposals and strategies. This became evident following the formation of the Carers (Recognition and Services) Act 1995, which as a result gave carers the right to request an assessment from social services based on their own need (NSF, 1999). Further development was then evident in the Mental Health National Service Framework (1999), which set standards within modernizing mental health services, with a view to promoting mental health and treatment, and put into place underpinning programs to support the delivery of these services. Incorporated into the framework is a standard, specifically for carers, intended to ensure that health and social services assess the needs of carers who offer support to individuals with a severe mental illness, where before such a service had at times failed. Since that time, further and ongoing recognition is evident.

Even more positively, the Department of Health published a document called *Developing Services for Carers and Families of People with Mental Illness* which aims to target local mental health support services for carers to ensure that carers gain access to resources and the support available (DoH, 2002). Throughout the country, support systems may vary in approach and quality, but their existence is compulsory. There is a wealth of information available for carers through a number of statutory and voluntary bodies, both locally and nationally, which can advise on carers' rights and other areas of need.

Under the Carers' and Children's Act 2000, a carer is entitled to a carer's assessment, even if the person they care for has not been or refuses to be assessed themselves. This assessment enables the carer to gain support in their own right (PDS, 2003). Within different areas of healthcare, responsibility for conducting an assessment can vary between disciplines, e.g., social worker, nurse, or independent service advisor. All of these professionals ought to be able to determine whether you as a carer are eligible for support within your role, what that support should be, and by whom it should be provided.

Role of the carer

A carer's role may encompass any number of tasks or responsibilities. This is dependent upon the service user's individual needs and the ability and limitations of the carer. For this reason there is no defined description as such. You will observe in Table 8.1 common recognized responsibilities in mental health, undertaken daily by many carers; however, the list varies and could go on for ever! A carer needs to be a "Jack of all trades" as well as having high levels of energy and compassion. Depending on the amount of time and support the carer offers, this can in turn affect the carer/service user relationship. Therefore it is important that all carers seek information regarding the mental illness affecting the person they care for. Having a greater understanding of what the individual sufferer experiences, the related symptoms and behaviors, and then the route to recovery, can help alleviate any misconceptions of mental illness. It can also reduce any unwelcome demands imposed on both the sufferer and the services supporting them. Furthermore this is an essential task to undertake as caring for a sufferer of a severe mental illness can be very stressful and challenging at times. Please read the relevant chapters of this book that introduce the concept of voices (Chapter 4), paranoia and unusual beliefs (Chapter 3), and, in particular, negative symptoms (Chapter 5) to enhance your current knowledge and understanding. It is the carer's understanding of mental illness that can dictate, and in turn impact on, any future course of action. This is in direct relation to what support they offer the service user, their approach and degree of involvement, and how effectively they work with agencies

Table 8.1 Common recognized responsibilities in mental health, undertaken by carers

- Monitoring medication
- Monitoring mental health
- Social contact
- Prompting all activities
- Taxi
- Housework
- Budgeting
- Laundry
- Making meals
- Prompting personal hygiene
- Assisting to dress
- Shopping

involved with the service user. Not forgetting, most importantly, maintaining their own health, which all helps the service user along the road to recovery.

Expressed emotion

The road to recovery can be a bumpy one, not just for the service user but the carer also, therefore it would be good for carers to be aware of different information that has moulded current practices and techniques used today in patient treatment. Research going back to the 1950s has found over the years that the environment the patient lives in can greatly affect their stability in mental health, level of social functioning, and prospect of recovery. This was initially recognized by a medical sociologist named George Brown from the MRC Social Psychiatry Unit in London, who observed that patients (diagnosed with schizophrenia) being discharged from (at that time) old large institutions, who returned to the family home, failed to progress as well and remain as long in the community, as those who moved on to live independently or within a residential setting (Brown, 1985; Brown et al., 1972). Clearly, families as such do not cause schizophrenia, therefore further research was undertaken into what may cause a patient to relapse within the home environment. The research undertaken explored the environment of individual patients who had relapsed, people within the patient's close environment, and their behaviors, attitudes, and responses leading up to the patient's relapse. Various dynamics highlighted a whole range of emotions being displayed, not necessarily by families or particular relatives but by "anybody" within the patient's close environment. The particular range of emotions expressed affecting the patients at that time were of high intensity and predominantly of a negative nature. These consisted of critical comments and hostility, and also some evidence of the carer presenting as over-involved; however, the latter appeared to have a lesser impact. These findings were monitored further. As patients were discharged home it was found that those who relapsed within a set follow-up period were those who went back to high levels of expressed emotion (EE) from the relative or others in the home environment, rather than those returning to low levels of EE. Further findings highlighted another main factor that affected relapse, this being the patient's continuous use of medication. Although this would appear obvious, again it was found that those within a low EE environment who did not take their medication stayed out of hospital for a longer period of time than those who did not take their medication but lived within a high EE environment (Barrowclough & Tarrier, 2001).

Summing up the aforementioned investigations, in order to make it easier to understand, the above findings emphasize the importance of good environmental dynamics and relationships for a sufferer with schizophrenia. The findings suggested that behaviors of a relative/carer, or activities within the service user's close environment that are of a negative nature, can create a heightened level of arousal for the sufferer of psychosis/schizophrenia (Barrowclough & Tarrier, 2001; Crisp, 2005). This heightened arousal is recognized as a form of stress. Like anyone who experiences a bad day and goes home feeling uptight or unhappy, a sufferer with schizophrenia or psychosis who experiences a difficulty in perception, attention, and thinking, can in turn experience an even greater level/awareness of their feelings/arousal/stress (Barrowclough & Tarrier, 2001). In essence, ongoing high levels of stress can be a predisposing factor to relapse for individuals diagnosed with a severe mental illness.

Getting the balance of a relationship right isn't easy. A carer may avoid a particular patient for many reasons, e.g., they don't know how to respond to them or may find them difficult to work with. As a result the carer may focus on other people's needs instead. This type of scenario could offer low levels or no levels of EE; however, this may result in the client being offered no support or attention at all. In turn, this could have a detrimental effect on the patient's thoughts, feelings, and emotions, which can affect their morale and motivation.

A carer may also try too hard in attempting to resolve any issues that may occur concerning the service user, e.g., insist on escorting them to the doctor's because they have been physically unwell, or insist on speaking on behalf of the service user because they don't talk very much (without realizing it is a negative symptom of schizophrenia). All the time the service user may think and feel differently to the carer and disagree with the carer's actions and comments; however, they do not feel confident enough to speak up to the carer who means well. Demonstrating emotional over-involvement can result in high levels of EE and affect the nature of the relationship and how the service user perceives the carer, e.g., controlling, frightening, or even a bully.

Questions to ask yourself

1. If the carers within the aforementioned studies were aware of Brown's findings, do you think they may have been more aware of the circumstance of the service user's environment and behaved or reacted differently towards them?
2. Have you ever considered if your everyday reactions or conversation could distress the person you care for?
3. Have you considered the environment the patient lives in and the behaviors of those around them?
4. Reflect on your answers and consider the following.
   a. Have these situations, experiences, or conversations ever been of a negative or critical nature?
   b. Can you recall a time when you were critical or negative to the service user to receive or provoke a similar response?
5. Did you think and react completely differently toward the person you care for, before gaining a greater understanding of schizophrenia and its related symptoms and experiences?

To assist you to answer the above questions, complete the work tool provided (see Table 8.2). The questions asked within the work tool are not designed to "point the finger of blame" but have been noted as common phrases that parents/carers use. The reason for this exercise is to attempt to raise your awareness of how general comments made by us all can affect an individual suffering from a severe mental illness. Tick the relevant boxes to the left of each example of comments, thoughts, and behaviors you have demonstrated. Follow the table across to gain a greater self-awareness of your behavior in order to consider how those identified behaviors could be interpreted by a sufferer of a severe mental illness.

Case studies

The following two case studies are examples to demonstrate how different approaches can affect EE and relationships. They also show how a sufferer of schizophrenia can interpret events that can affect or prove detrimental to their relationships, level of functioning, or mental health. The scenarios may

Table 8.2 Identifying expressed emotion

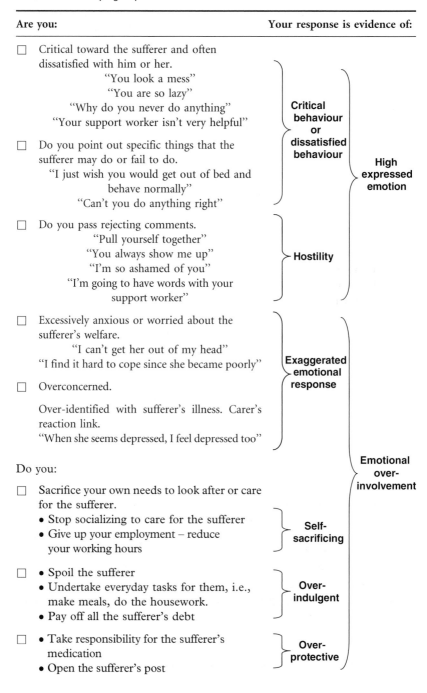

Are you:	Your response is evidence of:
☐ Critical toward the sufferer and often dissatisfied with him or her. "You look a mess" "You are so lazy" "Why do you never do anything" "Your support worker isn't very helpful"	
☐ Do you point out specific things that the sufferer may do or fail to do. "I just wish you would get out of bed and behave normally" "Can't you do anything right"	Critical behaviour or dissatisfied behaviour
☐ Do you pass rejecting comments. "Pull yourself together" "You always show me up" "I'm so ashamed of you" "I'm going to have words with your support worker"	Hostility
☐ Excessively anxious or worried about the sufferer's welfare. "I can't get her out of my head" "I find it hard to cope since she became poorly"	Exaggerated emotional response
☐ Overconcerned. Over-identified with sufferer's illness. Carer's reaction link. "When she seems depressed, I feel depressed too"	
Do you:	
☐ Sacrifice your own needs to look after or care for the sufferer. • Stop socializing to care for the sufferer • Give up your employment – reduce your working hours	Self-sacrificing
☐ • Spoil the sufferer • Undertake everyday tasks for them, i.e., make meals, do the housework. • Pay off all the sufferer's debt	Over-indulgent
☐ • Take responsibility for the sufferer's medication • Open the sufferer's post	Over-protective

Right-side brackets group: "Critical behaviour or dissatisfied behaviour" and "Hostility" → **High expressed emotion**. "Exaggerated emotional response", "Self-sacrificing", "Over-indulgent", and "Over-protective" → **Emotional over-involvement**.

appear pessimistic, but conversely aim to guide the carer to reflect on their identified thoughts and behaviors and then the possible consequence on both themselves and the service user. As stated above getting the balance right isn't easy, but more a road to discovery.

Case study 1

Jo first became unwell in her early 20s, but due to her passive quiet nature never demonstrated much evidence of ill health. She appeared to all around her to withdraw into her own world and isolate herself. Due to the warm nature of her family they accepted her behaviors. As time went on Jo stopped going out, and did not socialize. The family knew this was not normal but supported her. Jo deteriorated further. She went on to isolate herself more, and stopped communicating with particular family members who were unable to recognize that Jo was becoming increasingly unwell. Eventually Jo stayed in her bedroom for years, would not leave the room to eat, and appeared to lack the ability altogether to tend to herself and her personal hygiene. Throughout this time the family demonstrated unconditional love and support for Jo.

Once in her late 30s, Jo's family sought help from their primary care physician who involved mental health services. Following numerous home visits by services, Jo was detained in hospital under a section of the Mental Health Act, with a view to initiate treatment. On discharge from hospital, Jo returned to her parents' house.

Once again, Jo's relatives supported her with all her needs. At the age of 40, Jo once again lived mainly in her bedroom, had no responsibilities, and socialized only with her family.

Working together, both support services and Jo's parents assisted Jo to gain her own accommodation and furnish it, living independently. After Jo moved into the property, her mother and father moved in with her to make the transition easier. After two years they moved out; however, Jo's parents continued to stay over two or three nights a week. Their reason was to ensure that Jo did not feel lonely and also to ensure that she got up the following morning, took her medication, and attended the day care supports she had in place. This gave her parents the opportunity to clean the flat, tend to any washing, and ensure that Jo had plenty of food in the cupboards.

Jo's parents were never critical or hostile toward Jo in any way. Jo was mentally well-maintained and did not experience a re-admission into hospital. Jo did, however, rely heavily on her parents' support. Without their input Jo could not function independently in the home at all, and never left the home without her parents or support services.

Case study 2

Will recalled first feeling unwell in his early teens. He initially lived with his mother then went on to live independently soon after leaving school. Will lived within a strained environment where he loved all his family; however, dynamics were difficult. Both his parents had re-married and Will had two half-sisters. Will described living a stressful nomadic existence in order to maintain face-to-face contact with all his family members. Throughout this time he did not disclose to his family that he experienced difficulty thinking, and experienced strange thoughts. He eventually sought help from his primary care physician due to feeling low in mood. Soon after, he was referred to mental health services who felt that Will was experiencing a psychotic episode. Will agreed to take medication, which alleviated his symptoms; however, he continued to feel a little low in mood. Will's way of coping was to drink alcohol. Like most teenagers, Will would experiment with a full range of alcoholic beverages and failed to acknowledge the consequences of such in addition to the stresses of his current lifestyle, poor diet, lack of exercise, and existing mental health problem and medication.

Will maintained contact with mental health services and continued to take his medication as prescribed. Services attempted to reduce his medication in the hope that his psychosis would not return; however, Will immediately experienced difficulty sleeping and strange thoughts. Again, to help himself to cope, Will would drink alcohol, which perpetuated his problems further. As a result, Will's medication was changed. Throughout this time Will's mother re-married again and moved to a different area. This meant that Will would have to travel a considerable distance to visit her. Since his change in medication, Will had not remained as well as before and steadily deteriorated. While visiting his mother, Will became paranoid and believed people were chasing him, and he therefore carried a knife in order to protect himself. This resulted in Will drawing attention to himself, and he was arrested by the police. As a consequence Will was assessed and detained in hospital under a section of the Mental Health Act.

Throughout this time Will made it clear to services that he did not want either of his parents to be informed of his thoughts and behaviors (true experiences while psychotic) due to feeling embarrassed, a failure, and fear of rejection. As Will presented as lucid at times, and the rationale of his reasoning was sound, it was agreed that Will had the capacity to make such a decision.

Due to Will's length of stay in hospital, his tenancy was terminated on his flat to avoid any debt accruing; however, this meant that Will was then homeless. On discharge from hospital Will's mental health and level of functioning had deteriorated to the point where services felt Will would benefit from a period of care in rehabilitation in order for him to live independently again. Will was offered a place within a supported hostel to commence his rehabilitation within the area he was detained.

Throughout this time Will remained consistent, instructing services that he did not want his parents to know anything. In the meantime, Will's mother visited him on a regular basis. Each time she would ask Will questions regarding how he was feeling, what he was doing with his time, diet, exercise, even bowel movements, and what service support he had. Will found this very intrusive but feared his mother, and hence agreed with what she would say and do "for an easy life." Oblivious to his true feelings, Will's mother would organize activities for Will and prompt him to attend, in the hope that it would help him to get better, e.g., going for walks, attending bingo, and starting college.

Will found himself in a position where he was isolated, living in an unfamiliar area with no friends or other family members. He undertook all activities his mother organized for him, but eventually failed to maintain them due to the severity of his illness. Will's mother would then demand to know why Will had not undertaken tasks, e.g., daily living chores, attend college, etc., resulting in Will lying and denying having opportunities and supports in place, or he would say nothing in fear of disappointing her. As a result, Will would take himself off back to where he originally came from to visit his father, siblings, and friends. Will would then switch his mobile phone off to avoid his mother's calls. This resulted in services experiencing difficulty supporting Will. Throughout this time Will's mother would contact services and demand to know why Will hadn't progressed. Her level of concern would manifest itself in frustration and anger towards service support, resulting in poor relations and little collaboration in relation to care.

Now refer back to the questions on page 145 and see if you can relate them to the case studies.

Case study 1

Jo's parents demonstrated a number of different behaviors in order to support their daughter. Unbeknown to them, all of these were a form of EE recognized as emotional over-involvement; however, predominantly of a warm nature. Jo's parents may have thought more about the intensity of their support, and how much they were doing for Jo resulting in her lacking skills to undertake tasks independently, affecting her confidence, and motivation. Although the everyday reactions of Jo's parents did not lead to Jo experiencing any distress, in the event of them being unable to continue their current level of support, the consequences of such could result in Jo experiencing high levels of distress and inability to cope independently in the community. With a greater understanding of schizophrenia and related symptoms, Jo's parents may have accessed service support sooner and worked more closely with services to initiate social and functional support within the home and community. Jo's parents demonstrated an exaggerated emotional response, self-sacrificing behaviors, and overprotectiveness to the detriment of Jo.

Following a carer's assessment of need, Jo's parents built a good relationship with services. They endeavored to learn more about schizophrenia and worked closely with support services. As a result, Jo embarked on a new program of care utilizing a psychosocial approach, supported jointly by both services and her parents. Jo now follows a structured weekly program where she undertakes various activities, i.e., walking, gym, visiting places of interest, and attends clinics appropriately. She now shops with an escort, cleans her flat, and physically presents as socially acceptable. Jo maintains her own medication regime and has not experienced a second hospital admission. This was an example of carers gaining a balance in their involvement and relationship, demonstrating low levels of EE.

Case study 2

Will's mother demonstrated high levels of EE without realizing it, in expressing her concern and need to support her son. Will's mum may have considered an alternative approach to supporting Will rather than being dictatorial, which could have been perceived by Will as aggressive. This may have minimized Will's guilt for not progressing for his mother, resulting in poor self-esteem, low mood, and, in turn, Will avoiding her. As Will had not progressed to independent living, Will's mother may have considered the reasons why without pushing Will into feeling he ought to be living independently when clearly he was not ready. This resulted in Will feeling that he was letting people down and a failure. Will's mother expressed high levels of emotion of a negative nature, being particularly critical about service support to Will and demonstrating dissatisfaction and hostility toward both Will and services. She appeared extremely overprotective at times, and presented as preoccupied with Will's physical well-being rather than his mental well-being.

Once she accepted a carer's assessment, Will's mother was reluctant to be assessed and refused to answer relevant questions necessary to offer her support. The time offered in order to support Will's mother turned into an inquisition for the health care professionals, who were confronted and challenged with continuous questions regarding Will's well-being. Due to the overall dynamics of Will's family, his situation, and the poor relationship between his mother, service support, and himself, Will continued to struggle to progress. He remains in rehabilitation and continues to experience various symptoms of his illness, which possibly could be reduced. Will also continues to leave at every opportunity to visit his family in a different area, at times going without medication. The relationship between Will's mother and services remains strained to the point where Will continues to lie to his mother to avoid any conflict or being challenged, and as a consequence health care professionals are unable to liaise effectively with Will's mother. This example demonstrates how tense relationships can be between both carer, service user, and support services, resulting in difficulties and high EE.

Stress

Stress affects everyone at some point in our lives. We often view stress in a negative light but at times stress can have a positive effect, for example, some people perform or work better under pressure or the stress of a deadline. However, for the purpose of this chapter the former will be considered due to its association to ill health of both a physical and mental nature.

As previously discussed, stress can result in both a physical and psychological response. Referring back to the sufferer of schizophrenia or a carer who experiences difficulty coping, the pressures of ongoing exposure to stress can result in a heightened level of arousal. The effect on the individual will be dependent upon the amount of exposure one experiences and one's own level of vulnerability to stress. People simply have different coping abilities to one another.

Ever heard of the saying:

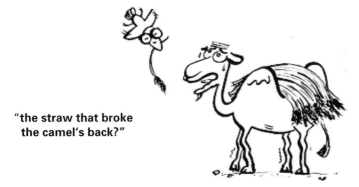

"the straw that broke the camel's back?"

When this occurs, stress can manifest itself in various ways, most commonly recognized by symptoms of anxiety or agitation (Zubin & Spring, 1977). On reflection, you may be able to recall a time while feeling stressed that you were experiencing difficulty sleeping or having no appetite. One may also recall feeling irritable and frustrated, and then experiencing difficulty concentrating or poor motivation (Williams, 2003). At times like this it would be fair to say that your level of tolerance for those around you has lowered, your response may be sharp and cold, and you may find yourself misinterpreting events or taking things personally or to heart that would normally not bother you. At times like this, our overall view and perception of everyday events are often quite negative.

If this is what you have experienced in the past, what makes a sufferer of a severe mental illness any different? Therefore one needs to bear in mind the consequences of a service user on the receiving end of a carer demonstrating stress, being potentially quite harmful. Refer back to Case study 2 when the carer expressed her anger to the service user regarding support services, she demonstrated hostile behaviors, and voiced comments of a critical nature. Although the comments were not necessarily in direct relation to the service user, the carer in effect pushed her frustrations toward the sufferer, which proved counterproductive. This in turn created fears and anxieties in the service user.

Gamble and Brennan (2000) talk about two forms of stress: ambient stress and life event stress. Ambient stress relates to everyday stressors of life, e.g., running late on a morning, disagreements with parents, or even paying a bill. Life event stress refers to events in one's life that create huge levels of stress, e.g., bereavement, separation, or losing your home. Referring back to the work undertaken by Brown in the 1950s and subsequent studies, an individual with a severe mental illness need not necessarily experience life event stress, but an increase in ambient stress. This could be enough to place the sufferer under pressure and make them more vulnerable to relapse or increase ongoing symptoms. When describing the effects of stress to people I work with, I ask them to imagine a pan simmering on the stove. We all simmer at different levels, and that's our level of vulnerability to stress (see Figure 8.1). When a stressful event occurs, our water level bubbles up (see Figure 8.2) then eventually it simmers back down again (see Figure 8.3). At times our water level may not simmer down before another stressful event occurs, resulting in the water level simmering at the top of the pan (see Figure 8.4). If one is unable to simmer down, the pan boils over (see Figure 8.5).

This could be understood as our breaking point. This is the point where we can no longer cope, experience poor health, or symptoms of anxiety – and for the individual who experiences a severe mental illness, an increase in their

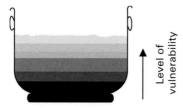

Figure 8.1 High levels of vulnerability lead to a lower ability to cope with stress

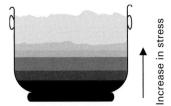

Figure 8.2 Increasing stress takes the user to the brink of experiencing psychotic symptoms

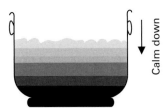

Figure 8.3 Reducing stress leads to psychosis being less likely

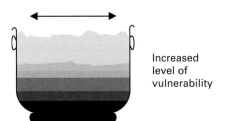

Figure 8.4 Further stress leads the user to the psychotic brink again

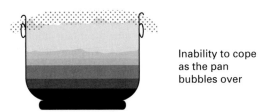

Figure 8.5 The stress leads to psychotic symptoms

symptoms, or even relapse in mental health. We need to be mindful that a service user's water level may simmer near the top of the pan most of the time, requiring little stress to bubble over!

If a carer explores events that have occurred with a service user leading up to their deterioration in mental health, the carer may be able to identify stressors. Together they can assist one another to a gain a shared understanding of the effects of stress and normalize thoughts and feelings in relation to the event.

Stress management

Everyone reacts differently to stress. As previously highlighted, the overarching stress response is of a negative nature, affecting one's mood and thinking, and resulting in a variety of feelings or symptoms, e.g., anxiety, frustration, anger, sadness, or sleep deprivation. All of these can alter how an individual reacts and what they do, therefore one needs to find a coping strategy that works for them to avoid such reactions. There are two ways of managing stress, firstly there is the obvious one, to take the stress away, depending on the nature of the problem itself. Referring to the stress I experienced in relation to my duties as a carer, I was able to ease the pressure at times by engaging the help of my friends and partner who would offer me practical support, i.e., purchase my grand-mother's groceries on my behalf and drop them off for me. My mother managed to alleviate her stress when my step-father would go into respite care for a week. These interventions worked in the short term; however, they do not necessarily reduce one's overall stress levels. For a carer of an individual with a severe mental illness, a route to reducing stress could be to seek similar help from support services enabling them to offer interventions that could reduce the problem causing the stressor itself, e.g., a change in medication. Or consider restructuring the patient's care to assist the carer. This could incorporate practical interventions involving a variety of resources, e.g., day services, or one-to-one support, which in addition to providing respite would also serve the purpose of introducing further stimulus to the patient (Kuipers, 1998).

The second way of managing stress as a carer could be to attempt to control one's negative emotions, thoughts, and behaviors linked to the stressor utilizing a cognitive approach. This could be achieved by undertaking your own personal interventions, e.g., relaxation, self-talk in order to compose one's self and rationalize concerns, or take time out to pursue hobbies and interests, in effect giving the carer the opportunity to simmer down as demonstrated in Figure 8.3. Also, a cognitive approach enables the carer to break the problem down. This will assist the carer to consider the dynamics of the problem and enable them to formulate causes or behaviors associated with the problem itself. In turn the carer establishes a greater understanding and is able to normalize the concern and undertake a problem solving approach, rather than reacting with a stress response. Problem solving need not be done in isolation but in discussion with the individual suffering from an illness. This also serves the purpose of assisting the carer to reappraise how they interpret the service user's behaviors and help modify their beliefs, hence enabling them to cope more effectively. Gaining a greater awareness of emotions linked to the service user's behaviors can help the carer in easing any feelings they may experience in relation to anger, guilt, or grief (Kuipers, 1998; MHA, 2006).

Cognitive approach to self-help

The term "Cognitive behavioral therapy" (CBT) or "cognitive approach" sounds complicated but can be quite simple. Cognitive behavioral therapy is based on the concept of how we think (cognitive) affects how we feel (mood) (Padesky & Greenberger, 1995). The approach aims to assist you to recognize negative or upsetting thoughts in order to challenge them. This can then help you to rationalize and normalize your thoughts. Thinking more realistically affects what we do (behavior), which enables you to look at the "here and now" and improve your state of mind, or at least can offer you some mental ease during stressful times (Williams, 2003).

Rationalizing a stressful moment or situation can be difficult at that particular time or at first, until you get used to using CBT techniques. It would therefore be easier at first to practice a formulation after the event/concern had occurred until you "get the hang of it." Formulation is a word we use to "set down" or "map out" what we are trying to break down into small parts. This then enables you to recognize the connection between the problem/ stressor and your, or the service user's, thoughts and reactions (Wilkinson *et al.*, 2003).

As mentioned throughout this chapter, a link between thoughts, feelings, and behaviors, is in itself a formulation that enables you to link your behavior back to your initial thoughts and related feelings (see Figure 8.6). Each part of the sequence affects the next part. As an example, to make it easy to understand, let's refer back to my own personal stressor discussed at the beginning of the chapter (see Figure 8.7).

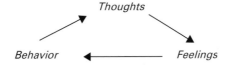

Figure 8.6 The relationship between thoughts, feelings, and behavior

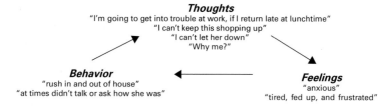

Figure 8.7 The relationship between thoughts, feelings, and behavior with examples

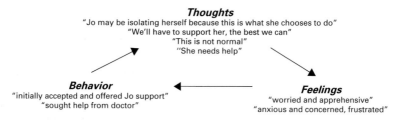

Figure 8.8 The relationship between thoughts, feelings, and behavior with examples from the case of Jo

> "My thoughts affected how I felt at that time, which affected what I did and how I did it."

On reflection on these events, I never considered how my behavior could have affected my grandmother's thoughts, feelings, and behaviors or evoked a response when I did have time to talk to her. The sequence developed further, and soon became a "vicious circle" of negative or distressing thoughts that increased my stress level.

Using the same formulation, refer to Jo's parents as discussed in Case study 1. (see Figure 8.8).

Using Table 8.3, recall your thoughts as a response to a problem or recent stressful event. Think carefully and write down what your thoughts were and how you were feeling at that time. Finally note down your response/ behavior as a result of your feelings.

Practicing the above will help you to "think on your feet," recognize unpleasant or negative thoughts you have previously experienced, and rationalize them. Identifying the above enables you to break the vicious circle and change other parts of the sequence. Whether it is the negative thoughts or the physical reaction that makes you feel worse, modifying parts of the sequence alters your overall responses. Again, using the same formulation and

Table 8.3 Practice table

Thoughts	*Feelings*	Behavior

(*Source:* Padesky & Greenberger, 1995)

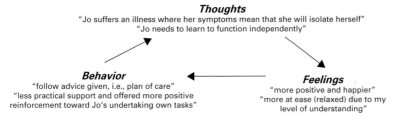

Figure 8.9 The relationship between thoughts, feelings, and behavior with further examples from the case of Jo

referring back to Case study 1, look at how changing either the thoughts or feelings affected the following parts of the vicious circle (see Figure 8.9). The overall impact of such induced a more positive response.

Another way to formulate is to use the "five area model" (Williams, 2001). Similar to the above sequence, the five area model can be applied in order to resolve various situations, support both a carer and service user to reduce stress, anxiety, and depression, as well as problem solve and improve your approach to positive thinking. The model provides a structured framework, as shown above, where its parts focus on current problems and reinforce the link between thoughts, feelings, and behaviors; however, it also incorporates

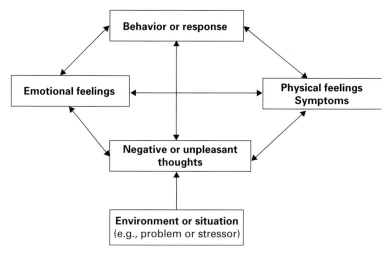

Figure 8.10 Five area model

additional core elements, i.e., emotions and the environment (see Figure 8.10). (If possible seek advice from support services to assist you to understand and practice the five area model.)

The five area model may appear a little complex at first, but it will be broken down into examples in order to make it easier to understand.

Look carefully and you can you see the similarity to Figure 8.6. As described earlier, our *thoughts* are our appraisal of our *situation* or current problems. These can then affect our *feelings* (as previously described in Figures 8.1–8.5) both *emotionally* and *physically*. Each area can then in turn affect our *behavior* or response to a problem.

This time we will refer to Case study 2 to demonstrate how the five area approach can be used to understand a situation. The list below describes parts of Will's situation under the headings of each core element.

1. *Environment* – Will was isolated, living in an unfamiliar area with no friends. Activities were arranged by mum that he did not want to do.
2. *Thoughts* – "I'm alone," "I miss my friends and sisters," "I don't want to go to the bingo," "I can't let my mother down."
3. *Emotional feelings* – Sadness and guilt, loneliness, trapped, weepy, under pressure.
4. *Physical feelings* – Problems sleeping, headaches, poor concentration, anxious (heightened level of arousal: tense, palpitations, sweaty, churning stomach, sickness).
5. *Behaviors* – Will would take himself off to visit other family members. Switch mobile off, demonstrating avoidance. Inability to progress due to above feelings and instability of mental health.

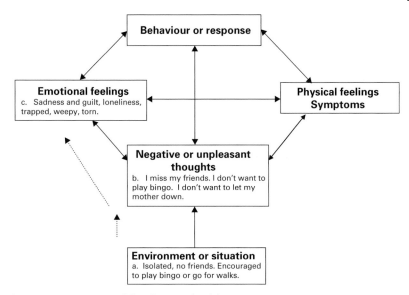

Figure 8.11 Five area model with examples (1)

Now we can use the five area model to formulate Will's situation, and gain a greater understanding as to why Will may have failed to progress at that time and behave in the manner he had. Following the dotted arrows in Figure 8.11, can you see the link connecting Will's situation to his thoughts? As a carer, do you think you might be able to identify similar related thoughts if you were aware of Will's situation? Would you be able to acknowledge the emotional feelings he may be experiencing as a result of his thoughts? The next stage of the formulation enables you to link Will's physical symptoms to either his emotions or thoughts (see Figure 8.12). At this point we have demonstrated a "vicious circle."

The final formulation (see Figure 8.13) links Will's behavior to his physical and emotional feelings as well as his negative thoughts. This time there are no dotted arrows to follow, as the solid arrows demonstrate that each core element within the formulation affects the others. For example, Will could experience numerous physical symptoms of anxiety that may exacerbate his emotional feelings, in turn, intensifying his negative thoughts and/or affecting his behavior or, even worsen, his mental health.

Now practice your own formulation using the approach above on the framework provided (see Figure 8.14). Rehearse a stressful situation or problem you have previously experienced in order to help you recall exactly what you were thinking and feeling. This will help you to understand your reactions and normalize your behaviors.

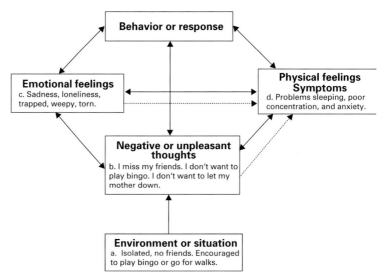

Figure 8.12 Five area model with examples (2)

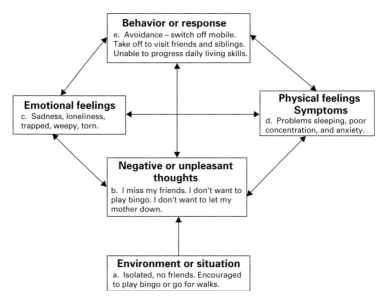

Figure 8.13 Five area model with examples (3)

Practicing the formulation can assist you to look at the broader picture in the event of stress or problem solving. Once you get the hang of it, you can begin to consider how and where within the framework you can break the vicious circle. This can be achieved by changing any component within the

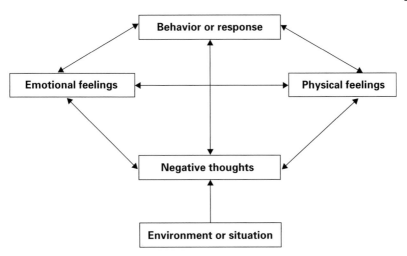

Figure 8.14 Blank template for five area model

framework facilitating an alternative response. For example refer to Figure 8.13; Will was experiencing poor sleep and poor concentration. Normalizing this problem, one could link emotional distress, i.e., weepy and low mood, as a response. If Will's sleep improved, it would be likely that his concentration would recover also. This would have a positive effect on both his physical and emotional well-being. Will or his carer may want to consider appropriate sleep hygiene in order to improve his sleep, e.g., regular exercise or relaxation techniques before retiring to bed.

Another example of attempting to break the vicious circle would be to consider Will's emotional feelings, i.e., sadness. Many people feel physically unwell when they feel low in mood, e.g., feel tired or experience aches and pains and therefore poor motivation. Physical symptoms as described earlier can lead to negative thoughts, which perpetuate the vicious circle further. Again Will or his carer may want to consider an appropriate action in order to improve Will's mood, e.g., encourage social interaction, suggest activities that Will would enjoy or have interest in, be positive, and give praise.

In summary, it is important to remember that our core elements, i.e., thoughts, feelings, and behavior can change and affect one another – therefore considering small actions can aid change in a positive way.

Cultural and religious aspects

Coming from a different cultural or religious background can sometimes add to the pressures of being a carer. For example, Asad's mother had recently come to stay with him from Pakistan as his father had passed away. Asad himself had suffered a relapse of his symptoms and had started hearing voices. His mother was convinced that he was possessed and wanted him to go to their holy shrine ("Dargah") and meet the priest for treatment. Initially Asad agreed with her, but as his symptoms deteriorated he finally contacted his care coordinator. A psychiatric outpatient appointment was arranged for Asad where his medication was increased and his care coordinator provided intensive support. He also arranged for Asad's mother to have carer support.

Initially, she was not happy with Asad's decision, but reluctantly agreed to receive help due to her inability to cope with her son's illness. In her sessions she disclosed that she missed the support of the family who were in Pakistan and worried about "what people would think if they found out." She also worried that somehow she was responsible for Asad's illness.

As Asad's symptoms improved, his mother started believing that medication might be helping and Asad continued to visit the shrine to pray, which made her feel happier. She also now believed that the services were not antireligion or culture.

Some worries and issues that carers face occur across cultures. However, some worries can be linked with the cultural and religious background of a carer. It is important to understand that either way, being a carer is stressful and any help and information should be welcomed.

Summary

This chapter has attempted to address some of the many issues highlighted by carers and observed by health care professionals every day; however, it merely scratches the surface in relation to what a carer could experience, think, feel, or need. It is therefore important to be knowledgeable and seek information regarding services available to support both yourself and the person you care for, and seek as much information as possible about the nature of the illness the sufferer experiences. It would be a good idea to always be aware of how your role impacts on not just the sufferer but yourself and others around you, and endeavor to sustain a low-stress environment in order to meet everyone's needs. This could be recognized and achieved by the following steps.

1. Acknowledging that being a carer can be stressful, therefore a carer needs to care for themselves first!
2. Aim to be aware of, and practice, the most helpful types of interaction, e.g., low EE.
3. Work with your relative/service user on the problems they wish to focus on, using the pertinent book chapters.

Most importantly, always ask for more support and guidance from experts when needed, whether this is in the form of practical or emotional help.

REFERENCES

Barrowclough, C. & Tarrier, N. (2001). *Families of Schizophrenic Patients. Cognitive Behavioural Intervention.* Cheltenham: Nelson Thornes Ltd.

Brown, G. W. (1985). The discovery of expressed emotion: induction or deduction. In J. Leff & C. Vaughn, eds., *Expressed Emotion in Families.* New York: Guilford Press.

Brown, G. W., Birley, J. L. T. & Wing, J. K. (1972). Influence of family life on the course of schizophrenic disorders: a replication. *British Journal of Psychiatry,* **121,** 241–58.

Crisp, A. H. (2005). *Every Family in the Land. Understanding Prejudice and Discrimination Against People with Mental Illness.* Worcester: GoodmanBaylis.

Department of Health (2002). *Developing Services for Carers and Families of People with Mental Illness.* London: Department of Health.

Department of Health (2006). Sharing mental health information with carers: pointers to good practice for service providers. *Continuity of Care. Briefing Paper.* London: Department of Health.

Gamble, C. & Brennan, G. (2000). *Working with Serious Mental Illness. A Manual for Clinical Practice.* London: Baillière Tindall.

Kuipers, E. (1998). Working with carers: interventions for relatives and staff carers of those who have psychosis. In: T. Wykes, N. Tarrier, & S. Lewis, eds., *Outcome and Innovation in Psychological Treatment of Schizophrenia.* Chichester: John Wiley & Sons Ltd.

Mental Health Association NSW Inc. (2006). *Caring for Someone with a Mental Illness.* www.mentalhealth.asn.au

National Service Framework (1999). *Modern Standards and Service Models. Mental Health.* London: Department of Health.

Padesky, C. A. & Greenberger, D. (1995). *Clinician's Guide to Mind Over Mood.* New York: Guilford Press.

Parkinson's Disease Society (2003). *Carer's Assessments. PDS Information Sheet.* London. www.parkinsons.org.uk

Wilkinson, G., Kendrick, T. & Moore, B. (2003). *A Carer's Guide to Schizophrenia,* 2nd edn. London: Royal Society of Medicine Press Ltd.

Williams, C. J. (2001). *Overcoming Depression. A Five Areas Approach.* Malta: Gutenberg Press.

Williams, C. J. (2003). *Overcoming Anxiety. A Five Areas Approach.* Bristol: Arrowsmith Ltd.

Zubin, J. & Spring, B. (1977). Vulnerability: a new view of schizophrenia. *Journal of Abnormal Psychology,* **86,** 260–6.

9

Staying well and managing setbacks

Shanaya Rathod

Overview

This chapter aims to offer the reader an understanding of how to prevent relapse by developing a relapse prevention plan based on their own likely stressors and individual relapse symptoms.

Chapter contents

- Case study 1
- How common are setbacks?
- What causes the setbacks?
- Biological, psychological, social: stress vulnerability factors
- Case study 2
- Managing stress
- Your high-risk times
- Your early warning signs
- Case study 3
- Cultural and religious aspects
- Case study 4
- Staying well plan
- Minor crisis plan/relapse drill
- Major crisis plan
- Summary

You have now reached a stage where you have managed to get some control of your symptoms. At this stage, focus will be on staying well and managing setbacks. Although it is possible that you may have difficulties in the future, there are things that you can do to minimize the chances of further difficulties. Understanding the difficulties and knowing your treatment options helps you to make better choices. This will mean that you do not need to be in constant fear of your symptoms returning. A very important aspect of working through this chapter is that we hope that you can reflect and learn through your own and other people's past experiences, and identify patterns and strategies.

You may have heard the word "relapse" being mentioned by various people. So, what is relapse? It can be explained as:

- worsening of distress or disability
- increasing of symptoms, or reappearance of symptoms
- a change in the nature of symptoms.

"Relapse" tends to mean a significant worsening in the person's condition or increase in symptoms, but this is very individual. In some people this will take the form of a temporary setback, though unfortunately in others it can become a "full relapse" – back to things being as bad as they ever were. We hope to minimize your chances of having a full relapse and show you ways that you can deal with minor setbacks so that they don't become a full relapse. In doing this, we hope to show you a staying well plan, to make you alert to your high-risk times, early warning signs, and also show you how you can help yourself if you spot these early warning signs.

Case study 1

I had a chest infection and struggled for days without medication, hoping the cough would go away. Finally my doctor started me on antibiotics and I started feeling better. After two days of being on the medication I had a sour taste in my mouth, and as I had been feeling better I decided to stop the tablets. Unfortunately for me, the cough became worse again within the next few days and I developed a temperature. I had to take time off work and repeat the course of antibiotics!

This example from experience confirms the fact that it is very easy to become complacent about treatment when one starts getting better, and to give in to the temptation of discontinuing treatment.

How common are setbacks?

From research, we know that most people with schizophrenia type illnesses, who have more than one episode of symptoms can have further episodes, and have similar symptoms for each bout of their illness. Sometimes even with the best combination of medication and other therapies, return of symptoms or relapse cannot be entirely prevented. This can give a feeling of being entrapped by the illness, and some people remain in constant fear of symptoms returning. Recognizing the symptoms early, and dealing with them, could prevent the symptoms from becoming severe.

What causes the setbacks?

Back in 1977, Zubin and Spring published their paper outlining the stress vulnerability model of mental disorder. The paper describes a simple principle that both stress and biology contribute to symptoms of illness.

You may have heard the professionals mention the term "biological vulnerability." This term refers to people who are born with, or who acquire very early in life, a tendency to develop a problem in a specific medical area. For example, some people have a biological vulnerability to developing diabetes or high blood pressure. Similarly, it is thought that people can have biological vulnerabilities to develop mental illness. The model explains that individuals have unique biological, psychological, and social strengths and vulnerabilities for dealing with stress (see Figure 9.1). When the stress becomes more than they can cope with, symptoms appear. Also, people's ability to deal with stress – their vulnerability – varies, so problems that one person may take in their stride might be enough to cause another person to become unwell.

Biological, psychological, social: stress vulnerability factors

Increasing coping skills or altering environmental factors (family, work, finance, housing, etc.) and sensible use of medication can reduce vulnerability and build resilience. Following are some things that have been found to increase chances of having a setback. We will explore them in some detail and discuss your thoughts about them.

Stopping medication

This is one of the most common reasons for a return of symptoms. Often, when well, people do not feel the need to continue with their medication. Some people also think that they will not be "normal" until they stop their medication.

• What are your views about continuing with medication?

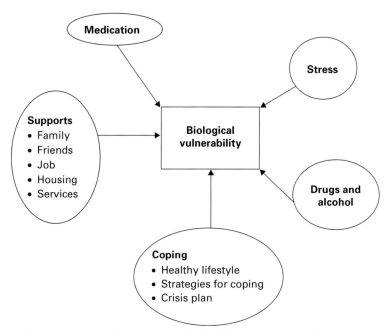

Figure 9.1 Factors that impinge upon an individual's biological vulnerability to psychosis

- Do you have any concerns about taking your medication long term? If so, what are they?

- Have you had any negative experiences through your treatment?

- How would things be different if you were not on medication?

- What would make you more confident about continuing your medication?

- Have you discussed your concerns with your doctor?

Case study 2

One young man with a serious mental health problem also had a cannabis habit. This caused him trouble on a number of fronts. Firstly, all concerned (including him) thought that heavy cannabis use was implicated in his original psychosis. Secondly, this young man was also very depressed and he really struggled to get up and do things. This was made worse by his cannabis use, and as a result he did little that would help him feel pleasure or a sense of achievement. Thirdly, this young man was living with his mum who tried hard to tolerate his smoking cannabis, but just could not stop nagging him about it from time to time. All of these factors increased the risk that this young man would experience stress, and this in turn increased the chances that he would have a setback.

Alcohol and illicit drug usage

Drugs and alcohol have a direct effect on the brain and cause return of the symptoms. Many people believe that the relaxing effect of drugs and alcohol helps with the symptoms, e.g., dampens the voices. What they do not know is that although at the time it feels like that, in the long term these substances affect the brain and make the symptoms worse.

- Do you use drugs/alcohol?

- What is your typical usage pattern?

- What does it do for you?

- Do you think your alcohol/drug usage affects your mental health?

Inactivity, isolating yourself, denying yourself pleasures

Often people feel that because they have suffered an illness, they do not deserve any pleasure and should not do any activity. Some people do not socialize, as they worry about their illness and what others might think about it.

- Do you do any of the above?

- How do you typically fill your day?

- Do your typical days contain opportunities for achievement and pleasure as well as the need to do chores?

- If not, what is stopping you?

- Would you like to identify some achievable goals and a plan to achieve them?

Missing sleep or meals

A regular and structured pattern to the day helps you to remain healthy.
- Do you miss meals or sleep?

- If so, why?

Managing stress

Stress is a part of day-to-day life, and everyone experiences it. How we cope with stress is important. Again, different people find different situations stressful. For example, going to work can be stressful for some whereas it could be stimulating for others. It is important to have reasonable expectations of oneself in life in order to avoid disappointment. A healthy lifestyle also helps to manage stresses, e.g., a good regular diet and exercise. Identify what stresses you most.

When stress occurs, it is helpful to have some strategies for dealing with it, so it will have a less harmful effect on you. Some helpful strategies are:

- talk to friends/family about your emotions
- use exercise
- use relaxation techniques, such as deep breathing, meditation, picturing a pleasant scene, or progressive muscle relaxation
- if you believe in a religion, use that to relieve stress
- think positive by saying things to yourself such as "I can do it"
- write your thoughts in a diary and discuss with your keyworker
- consider past coping strategies and use them
- use your hobbies.

Experiment with new ways of coping with stress. The more strategies you have, the better you can cope. Have you identified your coping strategies?

Your high-risk times

There are in all people's lives a number of high-risk times at which they may be more vulnerable to problems than at other times. These are likely to be the external events identified by yourself, which were linked with altered thoughts, feelings, or emotions. Patterns can be detected, such as:

- times of the year, week, or day when symptoms worsen
- meeting specific people (e.g., mother-in-law), especially if they are going to be present for a period, e.g., a holiday
- anniversaries – of becoming ill, of losses such as bereavements (including significant events in that person's life – birthdays, etc.), of admissions to hospital
- changes in medication
- watching a film, TV, or listening to music that is a reminder or trigger in some other way
- use of alcohol or drugs – or even use of these substances by others who they are with.

Can you think what your high-risk times might be?

Have you discussed these times with your family, carers, or therapist?

It might be helpful to make other people aware so that they might be able to increase their support for you. Is there anyone in particular that you think might be especially helpful to you at these times?

Your early warning signs

There is evidence to suggest that subtle changes in thoughts, feelings, and behavior precede a relapse and are characteristic for an individual. These are called early warning signs (EWS). These could be triggered by high-risk periods as identified above. Being aware of your EWS can alert you to the fact that things might not be right, so that you can take action. Try and remember your previous episode(s) of illness, especially the time before you or your carers realized that you were unwell. If you cannot remember everything yourself, you can discuss this with your carer or key worker for help.

Below is a list of common early warning signs:

- thoughts are racing and senses seem sharper
- having difficulty making decisions
- experiencing strange sensations
- feeling afraid of going crazy
- feeling sad, anxious, or restless
- feeling confused or puzzled
- feeling unable to cope with everyday tasks
- feeling irritable
- feeling like you do not need sleep
- speech comes out jumbled or filled with odd words
- neglecting your appearance
- not eating, not leaving the house
- drinking more, smoking more
- unable to sit down for long, behaving aggressively.

What were the thoughts, feelings, or behaviors concerning you at the time?

If you have one or even two of these symptoms it may indicate a problem developing. If problems develop, they can take two to four weeks before becoming serious. Because of this delay it is useful to keep an eye on your symptoms every week or two so you can do things to improve your chances of nipping things in the bud.

Case study 3

One young man was concerned about his EWS returning. For him, the most noticeable EWS was an interest in other women (he was in a steady relationship) and a tendency to use bad language. He was very keen to intervene early as he was determined not to jeopardize his relationship by these and similar behaviors. He had difficulty remembering to go through his EWS as a complete list, so we identified his "alarm bell" symptoms (swearing) and asked him to mentally check this on grocery day. This increased the chances that he would remember to do it regularly and not wait until the problem had developed into more of a crisis. He also shared with his partner what his plan was and we gave her a copy of his EWS and plans, so that she could gently remind him if there was an increase in swearing, which he might have overlooked. This worked well for him and he felt less concerned.

Cultural and religious aspects

Case study 4

A young man, originally from Zimbabwe and currently living in the UK, had suffered three episodes of psychotic symptoms. Each time a care plan was discussed, relapse signatures and EWS were identified, but during each episode the early symptoms were missed. He was well engaged with the services and was keen to identify signs and symptoms early. His friend attended during one of his appointments and casually commented that prior to his past two episodes, our young man had been talking about loneliness and wanting to return to Zimbabwe to be near his family. This was explored further and it turned out that this feeling was his actual EWS. This was incorporated into his care plan.

Relapse signatures are unique to individuals. Sometimes they are easy to identify but on other occasions they can be confused with normal thoughts and emotions, as in this example. When identifying your EWS, it is important to look at all options and possibilities. These could be dictated by your situation, culture, or religion among other things discussed above.

Staying well plan

This is a plan that aims to build upon what you have learned and has been helpful to you over the months and years. In many people there are things that have been found to help, and these should be entered onto a staying well plan. Things that people have typically identified as being helpful are shown below. Please go through the list and see which of these items has been helpful to you. Your personalized staying well plan might need to include these items and others especially relevant to you.

Helpful strategies

1. Taking my medication, even when I am feeling well and get it into my head I don't need it.
2. Avoid street drugs.
3. Keep myself busy.
4. Use my CBT strategies if I get paranoid thoughts, e.g., write them down and review the thoughts.

Plan A

Here is an example staying well plan, which we have labeled Plan A:
1. Continue my medication.
2. Try to keep myself busy, especially during the evening, making sure I do at least three pleasurable activities each day.
3. Each Wednesday do some "self-therapy" by checking my EWS, listening to a session tape, and reading my diary entries.
4. If there are more than three new symptoms, implement Plan B (minor crisis plan).

Minor crisis plan/relapse drill

This plan should be put into place if there has been an increase in your EWS. It is the type of plan mentioned in the example above as Plan B.

Plan B

1. Check that you have been taking your medication as it was prescribed. Many crises come about when people forget their medication or decide it's not needed because they are so well. If you have stopped taking your tablets, then start taking them again.

2. Plan activity levels that you are comfortable with. Find more things to keep you busy. If your mood is low, you will be tempted to do less, but you should in fact do more. Your activities should be planned, to ensure that you do things that give you a sense of achievement, and also things that have no skill but are pleasurable. These do not have to be expensive things. You might have to persevere with this for a few days on the assumption that these activities will take a few days to take effect.
3. Try to chat about your symptoms with people who you trust and who are helpful, such as professional people.
4. Check your EWS daily, and if they are reducing you can relax a bit, but if they remain the same or are increasing you might have to put into action the major crisis plan (see below).
5. Consider taking the phone off the hook for a while.
6. Use the TV and radio to provide background noise.
7. Use reasoning techniques. This means considering alternative explanations for the things you are bothered about, rather than an uncritical belief of your original thoughts.

    If you are hearing voices or comments, check that you can actually see the person's lips moving. If you need to clarify something with others, e.g., shop assistants, you should ask open-ended questions such as: "What did you say?" Avoid questions such as: "Did you just call me a . . . ?"

    When you have an unusual situation, ask yourself such questions as: "Is this likely?" "Is this possible?" "Would others (e.g., Dr Who) think this way?"
8. Keep your paranoid ideas or suspicions to yourself. Where possible you should avoid making decisions about people until you are absolutely certain. Where possible, try to get two or three sources of information before confronting people, regardless of how upsetting you think they might have been towards you. Be discreet to minimize the stigmatization that may occur if people think you are paranoid.

Example of Plan B

1. Check that I have done all of the things in my staying well plan.
2. Increase the amount of time spent doing pleasurable things, and reduce contact, if possible, with any unhelpful friends.
3. Monitor my EWS every two days until they start to reduce.
4. Drop in to the day center every day for a chat with my care worker.
5. Listen to the tape of rational responses from session 12 three times a day.
6. If my symptoms do not go away within a week, contact my psychiatrist and ask for an urgent appointment.

Major crisis plan

This plan should be put into place if your minor crisis plan has not brought about a reduction in EWS, or if you have had a major crisis.

1. Make sure that you have taken your medication as it was prescribed.
2. Make sure that you have been doing all of the things in the staying well plan, and all of the things in the minor crisis plan. Especially, make sure that you are getting enough sleep, not overdoing the alcohol, and that you keep yourself busy.
3. Seek expert help:

   Dr A . . .   on Tel: . . .

   Dr B . . .   on Tel: . . .

   Key worker . . .   on Tel: . . .

4. Once you have sought expert help, it is important to get on and try to help yourself. You can do this by continuing to do all of the things that you know will help to make you feel better, while avoiding things you know will make you feel worse.

Helpful actions

You might find it useful to list your helpful actions below.

1.

2.

3.

4.

Summary: staying well plan

Here is a list of strategies that you might find helpful to keep yourself well.

1. Keep stress down to a minimum. This might mean avoiding stressful situations, or at least trying to minimize these.

2. Make sure that you get enough sleep, as tiredness can make your symptoms worse. This is likely to be especially relevant at times, such as if you are physically unwell, have had an argument with a relative, or are worried or excited for some reason.

3. Continue with the medication. This means even when things are great, because it helps you to sleep well and helps to reduce stress. It also helps to protect you if you get additional stress in the future. Though you have concerns about side effects from your medication, most of the things you were concerned about are more likely to be part of the illness rather than from the medication.

4. Continue to avoid street drugs. These can cause the voices and paranoia to get worse.

5. Try to keep yourself busy. Work will obviously help with this, but even if you are not working or are sick, you should try and keep yourself busy.

6. Treat illnesses and infections with respect since they can affect your sleep and therefore your stress levels. If you have symptoms that can be treated, take some medicine, e.g., cough mixture. Consider involving your primary care physician if you are troubled by infections or other illnesses that might affect your sleep.

7. Avoid hangovers. This might mean reducing the amounts of alcohol you drink, or it might involve taking on extra fluids and pain killers before going to bed. Don't be tempted into using alcohol as a coping strategy.

8. Check your EWS weekly. It's worth keeping an eye on these signs so that you can do something early to reduce the chances of a major setback.

9. Be aware that you have a tendency to jump to conclusions and to scan the environment for evidence that people are talking about you or thinking badly of you. Remember that these things may not be true. It's better to keep cool and not to act suspiciously. Try and gather as much real evidence as you can before making any decisions about other people's intentions. Use the questions in this book to help you to gather realistic information.

Remember the cognitive therapy techniques in this book are best used with professional help. The techniques described are not dangerous, but at times things can become slightly worse before they begin to improve. Please seek advice from a mental health professional or primary care physician if you have any worsening in your mental health.

REFERENCES

Zubin, J. & Spring, B. (1977). Vulnerability: a new view of schizophrenia. *Journal of Abnormal Psychology,* **86**(2), 103–24.

Subject Index